Finding Serenity: A Guide to Living a Stress-Free Life

Dedication

In Loving Memory of my Late Mum, Naomi Murugi Maina

In the world of words, where pages come alive with stories and ideas, there is no tribute grand enough, no ink profound enough, to honour the memory of a beloved soul who has left an indelible mark on our hearts.

To my dearest Mum, Naomi Murugi Maina, whose radiant spirit and unwavering love continue to inspire me, this book is dedicated.

You were more than a mother; you were my guiding star, my source of strength, and the embodiment of grace. Your wisdom was boundless, your kindness boundless, and your love boundless still. You taught me the value of resilience, the beauty of compassion, and the art of finding serenity even in life's storms.

Though you are no longer with us in the physical realm, your presence lingers in every word, every thought, and every aspiration captured within these pages. It is through your enduring influence that I embarked on this journey to explore the pursuit of a stress-free life—a journey I am profoundly grateful to share with countless others seeking solace and wisdom.

As I pen these words, I am reminded of your unwavering belief in my potential, your encouragement to follow my passions, and your insistence on the importance of inner peace. It is your legacy of love and wisdom that guides the pages of this book, and it is your memory that fuels my determination to offer solace and guidance to those who, like us, have faced the storms of life.

Though you have embarked on a new journey beyond our earthly understanding, your lessons of love, strength, and resilience remain etched in my heart, a guiding light in the darkest of times.

This book, dedicated to your memory, is not just a collection of words but a testament to the profound impact you had on my life and the lives of countless others. Your legacy lives on, not only in these pages but in the hearts of all those who have been touched by your grace.

Thank you, Mum, for the immeasurable love, wisdom, and inspiration you shared with me and the world. As I share these words with others, I hope to honour your memory by helping others find their path to a more serene and fulfilling life.

Josiah Githinji

Table of Contents

- Introduce the concept of a stress-free life and its importance.
- Share a personal story or anecdote related to stress.
- Explain the purpose and structure of the book.

- Define stress and its various forms.
- Discuss the impact of stress on physical and mental health.
- Explain the difference between positive and negative stress.

- Help readers recognize the sources of their stress.
- Provide exercises and worksheets for self-assessment.
- Encourage mindfulness and self-awareness.

- Explore the connection between mental and physical health.
- Discuss the role of stress in chronic illnesses.
- Introduce relaxation techniques and their benefits.

- Define mindfulness and its role in stress reduction.
- Offer practical mindfulness exercises and tips.
- Share real-life success stories.

- Explain the importance of time management in stress reduction.
- Provide tools and strategies for effective time management.
- Share case studies of individuals who have transformed their lives through better time management.

- Discuss the concept of resilience and its importance in dealing with stress.
- Provide exercises and techniques for developing resilience.
- Share inspiring stories of people who have overcome adversity.

- Emphasize the role of nutrition, exercise, and sleep in stress management.
- Provide practical advice for making healthier choices.
- Include testimonials from individuals who have adopted healthier lifestyles.

- Explore a variety of stress reduction techniques, such as meditation, yoga, and deep breathing.
- Offer step-by-step instructions for each technique.
- Include personal anecdotes of how these techniques have transformed lives.

- Discuss the power of positive thinking in reducing stress.
- Provide tools for changing negative thought patterns.
- Share stories of individuals who have adopted a positive mindset.

- Explain the importance of social connections in stress reduction.
- Offer advice on building and maintaining healthy relationships.
- Share stories of people who have improved their lives through stronger social networks.

- Address common obstacles that readers may encounter on their journey to a stress-free life.

- Provide strategies for overcoming these obstacles.
- Include motivational quotes and anecdotes.

Chapter 12: Maintaining a Stress-Free Life

- Summarize key takeaways from the book.
- Provide a roadmap for maintaining a stress-free life.
- Encourage readers to continue their journey towards a stress-free life.

Conclusion

- Reflect on the transformation that readers can achieve by following the book's advice.
- Offer final words of encouragement and motivation.
- Provide resources for further support and learning.

Appendix

- Include worksheets, templates, and additional resources for readers.
- Provide a list of recommended books, websites, and apps for stress management.

Acknowledgments

Introduction: The Quest for a Stress-Free Life

In today's fast-paced world, the pursuit of a stress-free life often feels like an elusive dream. We wake up to the relentless demands of our daily routines, battling deadlines, navigating traffic, managing responsibilities, and striving for success. As our lives become increasingly complex, stress has woven itself into the very fabric of our existence, like an unwelcome guest who refuses to leave.

But what if I told you that living a stress-free life is not just a distant fantasy? What if I shared with you the secrets to reclaiming your serenity, one step at a time? In the pages of this book, we embark on a transformative journey, exploring the profound concept of a stress-free life and unravelling its profound importance.

The Weight of Stress

Stress, in its many forms, can weigh us down like an anchor, preventing us from sailing smoothly through life's waters. It affects not only our mental well-being but also our physical health. The relentless pressure of stress can lead to anxiety, depression, insomnia, and a myriad of other health issues. It can chip away at our relationships, hinder our creativity, and stifle our potential.

Yet, the paradox of modern life is that while stress is ubiquitous, so too is our desire to escape its clutches. We long for moments of peace, for a respite from the turmoil, for a life where joy and fulfillment take precedence over worry and exhaustion.

The Promise of a Stress-Free Life

A stress-free life is not about escaping challenges or seeking an existence devoid of responsibility. It is about mastering the art of managing stress in a way that allows you to thrive, not just survive. It's about reclaiming your power, your happiness, and your inner calm.

Imagine waking up each morning with a sense of purpose, unburdened by the weight of anxiety. Envision facing life's inevitable challenges with resilience and grace, confident in your ability to navigate them. Picture yourself nurturing deep and meaningful relationships, free from the distractions of stress-induced turmoil. This is the promise of a stress-free life.

Why This Book Matters?

The importance of this journey cannot be overstated. It's about more than just feeling better; it's about living better. It's about reclaiming your life from the clutches of stress and rediscovering the joy that often gets buried beneath life's demands.

Throughout the pages that follow, we will explore the roots of stress, identify its insidious sources, and equip you with a treasure trove of tools and strategies to combat it. We'll delve into the science of stress and the art of mindfulness, time management, and positive thinking. We'll share inspirational stories of individuals who have transformed their lives by embracing these principles.

So, whether you're feeling overwhelmed by the demands of your career, weighed down by personal struggles, or simply seeking a more serene and meaningful existence, this book is your guide to reclaiming your life, one stress-free moment at a time. The journey won't always be easy, but it will be profoundly rewarding, for in the pursuit of a stress-free life, you'll discover not only peace but also the limitless potential within yourself. Welcome to the adventure of a lifetime.

Preface: The Pursuit of a Stress-Free Life

Welcome to the pages of "Stress-Free Life," a journey that begins with a simple yet profound question: What if life didn't have to be so stressful?

In the hustle and bustle of our modern world, stress has become a ubiquitous companion, lurking in the shadows of our daily lives. It manifests in our workplaces, seeps into our homes, and even infiltrates our moments of solitude. But is this the life we truly desire? Is this the legacy we wish to leave for ourselves and those we love?

The idea for this book was born out of a personal revelation. Like many, I found myself caught in the relentless grip of stress, juggling the demands of a career, family, and personal aspirations. I watched as the hours slipped away, and I yearned for a life where stress was not the ruler of my existence.

Through countless hours of research, self-reflection, and conversations with individuals who had successfully tamed the stress beast, I discovered that the pursuit of a stress-free life is not only attainable but also transformative. It is a journey filled with valuable lessons, small victories, and profound realizations.

In the pages that follow, we will embark on this journey together. We will explore the roots of stress, confront its formidable presence, and equip ourselves with the tools and strategies needed to live life on our terms. This book is not a promise of a stress-free existence, for such a utopia does not exist. Rather, it is a roadmap to a life where stress no longer holds dominion.

As you turn these pages, you'll encounter stories of triumph over adversity, practical exercises to build resilience, and insights that can reshape your perspective on stress. You'll discover the power of mindfulness, the art of time management, and the profound impact of positive thinking. Most importantly, you'll find that a stress-free life is not a distant dream but a tangible reality within your grasp.

This book is for you, whether you're a corporate executive navigating the pressures of the boardroom, a caregiver seeking balance in a hectic schedule, a student struggling with the weight of expectations, or simply someone who yearns for a more serene and fulfilling life. It is my hope that the wisdom shared within these pages will inspire you, empower you, and guide you on your journey to a life less encumbered by stress.

The path ahead may be challenging at times, but remember this: the pursuit of a stress-free life is not about avoiding difficulties but about mastering them. It's about embracing life's challenges with a clear mind, a courageous heart, and an unwavering belief in your own resilience.

So, dear reader, I invite you to join me on this transformative journey. Let us embark together on the quest for a stress-free life—one page, one chapter, and one step at a time.

Chapter 1:

An Unexpected Encounter with Stress: A Personal Tale

Stress, in all its various forms, has a way of creeping into our lives when we least expect it. It's a silent intruder, lurking in the shadows until it decides to reveal itself. Allow me to share a personal story that underscores the unpredictable nature of stress and its impact on our lives.

Several years ago, I found myself in a job that I loved but that was increasingly demanding. I had a passion for my work, and I thrived on the challenges it presented. However, I didn't realize that I was gradually becoming a victim of my own ambition.

One sunny morning, as I was rushing to a crucial meeting, I received an urgent call. It was my elderly neighbour, Madam Wairimu. She had fallen and needed immediate assistance. Without hesitation, I abandoned my carefully planned schedule and rushed to her aid. The following hours were a blur of hospital corridors, medical jargon, and concerned discussions with doctors.

In the days that followed, Madam Wairimu's health remained fragile, and I found myself juggling my demanding job with the responsibilities of caregiving. It was a precarious balancing act, and stress began to weave its insidious web around me. The pressure of deadlines at work collided with the emotional toll of caring for my neighbor, and I was caught in the crossfire.

As the days turned into weeks, I noticed changes in myself that I had never anticipated. I struggled to sleep, my once-healthy diet took a backseat to quick and unhealthy meals, and my normally calm demeanour was replaced by irritability and anxiety. Stress, it seemed, had claimed a firm grip on my life.

It was during this challenging period that I learned some valuable lessons about stress. I realized that it wasn't just the external pressures at work or the demands of caregiving that were causing my distress; it was my response to those pressures. I had neglected to take care of my own well-being in the process of caring for others and pursuing my career goals.

This experience was a wake-up call, prompting me to reevaluate my priorities and seek a healthier balance in my life. It taught me that stress can infiltrate our lives in unexpected ways, and it's essential to be mindful of its presence and its impact.

In the chapters that follow, we'll delve deeper into the understanding of stress, its various forms, and how we can proactively manage it. My hope is that by sharing my personal encounter with stress, you'll see that you are not alone in facing this formidable adversary and that there are strategies and techniques to regain control over your life and find serenity even in the midst of life's storms.

Introduction: The Purpose and Structure of this Book

In the quest for a stress-free life, having a clear roadmap and a sense of purpose is essential. This book is designed to provide you with precisely that—a roadmap to living a life that is less burdened by stress and a profound sense of purpose that stems from reclaiming your inner peace.

Purpose of the Book:

The primary purpose of this book, "Stress-Free Life," is to empower you to take control of the stress in your life, no matter its source or intensity. It's about helping you transform stress from an overwhelming adversary into a manageable companion. Through knowledge, practical exercises, and inspiring stories, this book aims to:

1. **Educate:** You will gain a deep understanding of stress, its various forms, and its impact on your physical and mental well-being. Knowledge is the first step toward empowerment.
2. **Empower:** Armed with insights and strategies, you will learn how to identify and manage your stressors effectively. You'll develop resilience and the ability to face challenges with confidence.

Inspire: Throughout the book, you will encounter real-life stories of individuals who have overcome significant stress and adversity.

Understanding Stress

The Invisible Weight: Unveiling the Mysteries of Stress

Stress—such a simple word, yet it carries the weight of a thousand burdens. It's a term we throw around casually, often underestimating its power and prevalence. But before we embark on our journey to live a stress-free life, we must first understand our adversary. In this chapter, we will delve into the intricacies of stress, exploring its forms, its origins, and its impact on our lives.

Defining Stress:

At its core, stress is the body's natural response to a demand or threat. It's the alarm system that kicks in when we perceive danger, whether real or imagined. This response triggers a cascade of physiological changes—increased heart rate, rapid breathing, heightened alertness—that prepare us to confront the perceived threat. This is known as the "fight or flight" response.

But here's the catch: stress isn't inherently negative. In fact, there are two primary types of stress:

1. **Eustress:** This is positive stress, the kind that motivates us to perform well in challenging situations. It's the excitement before a big presentation, the adrenaline rush during a thrilling adventure, or the nervousness before a significant life event. Eustress can be invigorating and lead to personal growth.
2. **Distress:** This is the negative stress we often associate with the term. It's the chronic worry, the overwhelming pressure, and the daily grind that feels like an insurmountable burden. Distress can have detrimental effects on our mental and physical health.

The Many Faces of Stress:

Stress is not a one-size-fits-all phenomenon. It comes in various forms, each with its unique characteristics and impact:

1. **Acute Stress:** This is the short-term stress we experience when faced with an immediate threat or challenge. It's the kind that spikes during

a traffic jam or a sudden work deadline. While it can be uncomfortable, acute stress typically subsides once the situation is resolved.

2. **Chronic Stress:** This is the relentless, long-term stress that can permeate every aspect of our lives. It may stem from ongoing financial troubles, a toxic work environment, or the strains of caregiving. Chronic stress can lead to severe health issues if left unchecked.

3. **Environmental Stress:** Stressors in our physical surroundings, such as noise pollution, overcrowding, or a chaotic living space, can contribute to our overall stress levels.

4. **Emotional Stress:** Emotional turmoil, like grief, relationship problems, or personal setbacks, can be a significant source of stress.

5. **Cognitive Stress:** This form of stress is rooted in our thought patterns—negative self-talk, excessive worry, and perfectionism can create chronic cognitive stress.

The Impact of Stress:

Understanding stress also means recognizing its far-reaching consequences:

- **Physical Health:** Chronic stress can lead to a range of physical health issues, including heart disease, high blood pressure, digestive problems, and weakened immune function.
- **Mental Health:** Stress is a major contributor to conditions like anxiety disorders, depression, and burnout.
- **Behavioral Changes:** Stress can influence our behaviors, leading to unhealthy coping mechanisms such as overeating, substance abuse, or withdrawal from social activities.
- **Interpersonal Relationships:** Stress can strain relationships, as heightened emotions and irritability may affect how we interact with loved ones.

The Purpose of Understanding Stress:

The purpose of this chapter is not to overwhelm you with the enormity of stress but to arm you with knowledge. Understanding stress is the first step in conquering it. By recognizing its various forms and the impact it has on your life, you'll be better equipped to navigate the journey ahead.

In the chapters to come, we will delve deeper into strategies for identifying and managing your specific stressors. We will explore the mind-body connection, the power of mindfulness, and the art of finding serenity amidst life's demands. Remember, the pursuit of a stress-free life begins with understanding the enemy—and that's precisely what we've done here.

Defining Stress and Its Various Forms

Stress is a complex and multifaceted phenomenon that affects individuals physically, emotionally, and mentally. It is the body's natural response to a demand or threat, and it can manifest in various ways. Here, we'll define stress and explore its various forms:

Definition of Stress:

Stress is the body's physiological and psychological response to a perceived threat or demand. When faced with a challenging situation, the body activates its "fight or flight" response, a series of physical and mental changes designed to help us confront or escape from the perceived threat.

Now, let's delve into the various **forms of stress:**

1. **Eustress:** This is positive stress, often referred to as "good stress." Eustress is characterized by feelings of excitement, motivation, and engagement. It arises from situations where the challenge is manageable and can lead to personal growth and achievement. Examples include starting a new job, preparing for a competition, or planning a wedding.
2. **Distress:** This is the negative form of stress, the one most commonly associated with the term "stress." Distress arises when individuals face excessive or overwhelming demands that they perceive as threatening. It can manifest in physical and emotional symptoms and can have adverse effects on health and well-being. Examples include chronic work-related pressures, financial problems, or the loss of a loved one.

3. **Acute Stress:** Acute stress is short-term and often occurs in response to a specific event or situation. It is a natural response to immediate challenges and typically subsides once the situation is resolved. For example, the stress experienced during a near-miss accident or before a big presentation is acute stress.

4. **Chronic Stress:** Chronic stress is long-term and persistent. It results from ongoing, unrelenting stressors that individuals perceive as beyond their control. Chronic stress can lead to a range of physical and mental health issues, including heart disease, anxiety disorders, and depression. Examples include prolonged work-related stress, financial instability, or a toxic living environment.

5. **Environmental Stress:** This form of stress is related to the physical environment in which an individual lives or works. It can result from factors like noise pollution, overcrowding, or exposure to environmental toxins. Environmental stress can contribute to overall stress levels and affect well-being.

6. **Emotional Stress:** Emotional stress arises from intense emotional experiences, such as grief, relationship conflicts, or personal setbacks. It can lead to emotional turmoil and may have physical manifestations like headaches or gastrointestinal distress.

7. **Cognitive Stress:** Cognitive stress is rooted in our thought patterns and mental processes. It often involves negative self-talk, excessive worry, and rumination. Cognitive stress can perpetuate anxiety and contribute to chronic stress.

8. **Interpersonal Stress:** This type of stress originates from challenges in interpersonal relationships, whether with family members, friends, or colleagues. Interpersonal stressors, such as conflicts or strained relationships, can significantly impact an individual's well-being.

Understanding these various forms of stress is essential because it allows individuals to recognize and address the specific stressors in their lives. Each form may require different strategies for management and coping. In the chapters that follow, we will explore techniques and practices to help you manage stress effectively, regardless of its form.

The Impact of Stress on Physical and Mental Health

Stress is not just an uncomfortable feeling; it can have profound and far-reaching effects on both physical and mental health. Understanding these impacts is crucial because it highlights the importance of managing and mitigating stress in our lives.

Physical Health Impact:

1. **Cardiovascular Problems:** Chronic stress can lead to increased blood pressure, which, over time, can contribute to hypertension (high blood pressure). Hypertension is a major risk factor for heart disease, stroke, and other cardiovascular conditions.
2. **Immune System Suppression:** Prolonged stress can weaken the immune system, making the body more susceptible to infections and illnesses. This weakened immunity can result in more frequent colds, flu, and other infections.
3. **Digestive Issues:** Stress can disrupt normal digestive processes, leading to symptoms such as indigestion, acid reflux, irritable bowel syndrome (IBS), and even ulcers. Chronic stress may contribute to the development of gastrointestinal disorders.
4. **Weight Gain:** Stress can trigger overeating or the consumption of unhealthy comfort foods, leading to weight gain. The body's response to stress includes the release of cortisol, a hormone associated with increased appetite and fat storage, particularly in the abdominal area.
5. **Sleep Disorders:** Stress and anxiety can interfere with sleep patterns, leading to insomnia or poor-quality sleep. Sleep deprivation, in turn, can exacerbate stress and negatively impact overall health.
6. **Muscle Tension and Pain:** Stress often manifests as muscle tension, which can lead to headaches, migraines, and other forms of chronic pain, such as tension-type or neck and shoulder pain.
7. **Skin Problems:** Stress can exacerbate skin conditions like acne, psoriasis, and eczema. It can also contribute to the premature aging of the skin and delay wound healing.

Mental Health Impact:

1. **Anxiety Disorders:** Chronic stress is a major contributor to the development and exacerbation of anxiety disorders, including generalized anxiety disorder (GAD), panic disorder, and social anxiety disorder.
2. **Depression:** Prolonged or severe stress can lead to depression. Stress-related depression is characterized by persistent feelings of sadness, hopelessness, and a loss of interest or pleasure in activities.
3. **Post-Traumatic Stress Disorder (PTSD):** Exposure to significant trauma or stressors can lead to PTSD, a condition characterized by flashbacks, nightmares, and severe anxiety in response to triggers associated with the traumatic event.
4. **Substance Abuse:** Some individuals turn to alcohol, drugs, or other substances as a way to cope with stress. Substance abuse can exacerbate mental health issues and lead to addiction.
5. **Cognitive Impairment:** Chronic stress can impair cognitive functions such as memory, attention, and decision-making. This can hinder academic or work performance and contribute to feelings of frustration.
6. **Social Isolation:** Stress can lead to withdrawal from social activities and relationships, increasing feelings of loneliness and exacerbating mental health issues.
7. **Suicidal Thoughts:** In severe cases, chronic stress, depression, and anxiety can lead to suicidal thoughts or behaviours. It's essential to seek professional help if you or someone you know is experiencing such thoughts.

Understanding the profound impact of stress on physical and mental health underscores the importance of proactive stress management. Effective stress reduction techniques, such as mindfulness, exercise, and seeking social support, can help mitigate these adverse effects and promote overall well-being. Additionally, if you or someone you know is struggling with chronic stress or its mental health consequences, seeking the guidance of a healthcare professional is essential for appropriate diagnosis and treatment.

Positive Stress (Eustress) vs. Negative Stress (Distress)

Stress is a natural and adaptive response that the body and mind employ to deal with various challenges and demands in life. It's important to recognize that not all stress is harmful; in fact, there are two primary categories of stress, each with distinct characteristics and effects:

1. Positive Stress (Eustress):

Characteristics:

- **Motivating:** Eustress is often associated with feelings of excitement, anticipation, and engagement. It can be a driving force that motivates you to take action and achieve your goals.
- **Short-Term:** Eustress is typically short-lived and results from manageable challenges or situations. It arises in response to events or circumstances that you perceive as positive or beneficial.
- **Enhancing Performance:** Eustress can improve cognitive function and performance. It can help you stay focused, alert, and energized, enhancing your ability to tackle tasks and meet deadlines.

Examples of Eustress:

- Preparing for a wedding or a big celebration.
- Starting a new job or embarking on a new career.
- Engaging in exciting physical activities, such as skydiving or extreme sports.
- Pursuing personal goals or passions that you're enthusiastic about.

2. Negative Stress (Distress):

Characteristics:

- **Overwhelming:** Distress is often characterized by feelings of overwhelm, anxiety, and unease. It arises from situations or demands that you perceive as threatening, challenging, or beyond your ability to cope.
- **Chronic or Prolonged:** Unlike eustress, distress can be persistent and long-lasting. It may result from ongoing or unrelenting stressors,

such as financial difficulties, work-related pressures, or chronic health issues.

- **Detrimental Effects:** Distress can have adverse effects on physical and mental health. It can lead to symptoms such as irritability, mood swings, fatigue, and physical health problems, including heart disease and digestive issues.

Examples of Distress:

- Coping with the loss of a loved one.
- Experiencing chronic financial problems or job insecurity.
- Facing ongoing relationship conflicts or personal crises.
- Dealing with the demands of caregiving for a loved one with a chronic illness.

Key Differences:

1. **Perception:** The primary distinction between eustress and distress is how you perceive the stressor. Eustress arises from situations you perceive as positive or exciting, whereas distress stems from situations that are perceived as negative, challenging, or overwhelming.
2. **Duration:** Eustress is typically short-term and often associated with acute situations, whereas distress can be chronic and persist over an extended period.
3. **Effect on Well-Being:** Eustress can enhance well-being, motivation, and performance, while distress, if not managed effectively, can have detrimental effects on physical and mental health.
4. **Response:** Eustress often leads to a "challenge" response, where you feel motivated to take action. In contrast, distress can trigger a "threat" response, characterized by anxiety and the activation of the body's stress response systems.

Understanding the difference between these two forms of stress is essential because it allows individuals to recognize when stress can be a positive motivator and when it requires effective coping strategies to prevent its negative impact on well-being. While eustress can enhance life experiences and achievements, distress calls for proactive stress management techniques to minimize its adverse effects on health and overall quality of life.

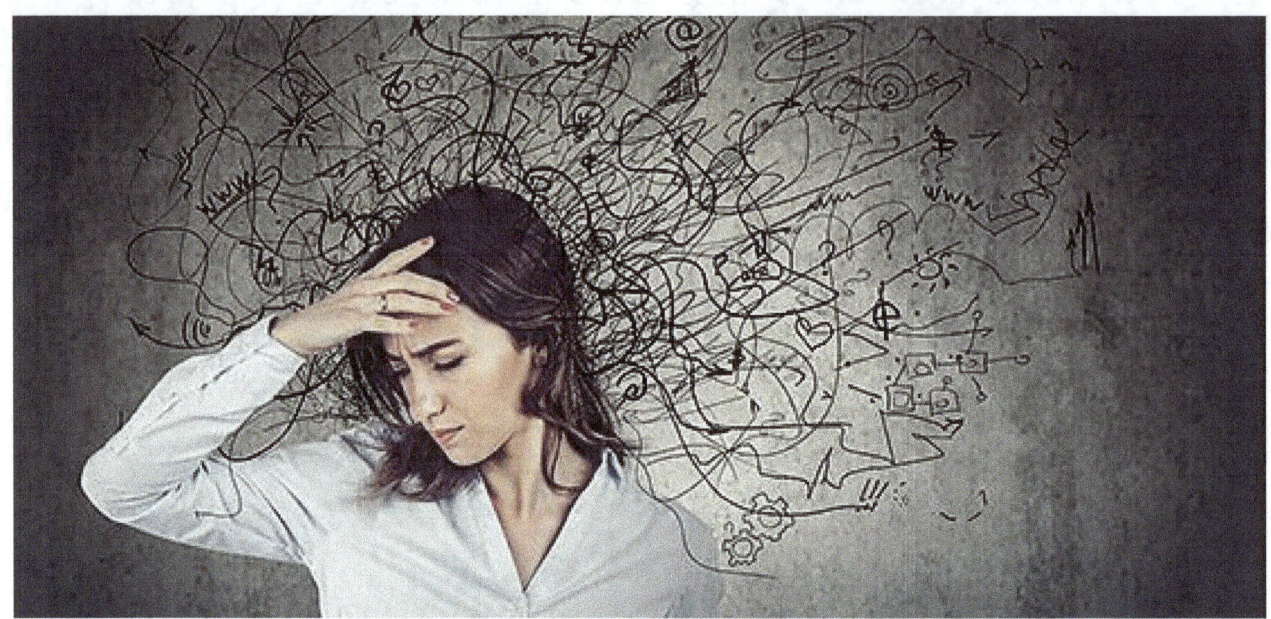

Stress That generate severe headache!

Chapter 2

Unveiling the Hidden Culprits:

In the pursuit of a stress-free life, one of the most crucial steps is understanding the specific stressors that affect you personally. Stressors are like shadows, often lurking in the background of our lives, subtly sapping our energy and well-being. In this chapter, we will embark on a journey of self-discovery to uncover and shed light on the sources of your stress.

The Importance of Identifying Stressors:

Why is it essential to identify your stressors? Because, as the saying goes, "knowing is half the battle." When you can pinpoint the root causes of your stress, you gain a significant advantage in managing and mitigating it. By understanding your stressors, you can:

- **Take targeted action:** You can develop strategies and coping mechanisms specifically tailored to address the sources of your stress.
- **Prevent overwhelm:** Identifying stressors allows you to tackle them proactively, preventing them from accumulating and becoming overwhelming.
- **Enhance self-awareness:** Recognizing your stressors fosters self-awareness, empowering you to make informed choices about your lifestyle and priorities.

Exploring Different Categories of Stressors:

Stressors can manifest in various areas of your life. Some common categories of stressors include:

1. **Work-Related Stressors:** These may include heavy workloads, tight deadlines, conflicts with colleagues or supervisors, job insecurity, or a lack of work-life balance.
2. **Financial Stressors:** Concerns about debt, bills, financial instability, or the cost of living can be significant stressors.
3. **Relationship Stressors:** Strained relationships with family members, friends, or romantic partners can contribute to emotional stress.

4. **Health-Related Stressors:** Coping with chronic illnesses, managing health conditions, or dealing with medical bills can be highly stressful.
5. **Life Transitions:** Major life changes such as moving, getting married, having a baby, or experiencing the loss of a loved one can be sources of stress.
6. **Personal Stressors:** These may include perfectionism, negative self-talk, or unrealistic personal expectations.

Identifying Your Personal Stressors:

To identify your stressors effectively, consider the following steps:

1. **Self-Reflection:** Take time to reflect on recent periods of stress in your life. What were the circumstances or events that triggered stress during those times?
2. **Journaling:** Keeping a stress journal can help you track stressors over time. Record stressful incidents, your emotional responses, and any physical symptoms.
3. **Self-Assessment:** Use self-assessment tools or questionnaires designed to identify stressors in different areas of your life, such as work, relationships, or personal habits.
4. **Seek Feedback:** Sometimes, friends, family, or colleagues can provide insights into stressors you may not be fully aware of. Don't hesitate to seek their input.
5. **Professional Guidance:** If you're struggling to identify your stressors or believe they may be related to deeper issues, consider consulting a mental health professional or counsellor for guidance.

The Road Ahead:

As you uncover your stressors, remember that this process is an essential step toward regaining control over your life. The next chapters will delve deeper into strategies for managing and mitigating the specific stressors you identify. Whether it's work-related stress, financial worries, or personal challenges, there are effective tools and techniques available to help you on your journey to a more stress-free life.

Identifying your stressors is like shining a light into the darkest corners of your life, revealing the sources of your discomfort and paving the way for transformative change. As we move forward, you'll discover that with knowledge and proactive measures, even the most entrenched stressors can be conquered.

Recognizing the sources of stress in your life is a crucial step towards effective stress management and living a more balanced, fulfilling life. Here are some strategies and tips to help readers recognize and identify their personal stressors:

1. Self-Reflection:

Encourage yourself to take time for self-reflection. Set aside quiet moments to contemplate your thoughts, emotions, and daily experiences. Journaling can be an effective tool for self-reflection. Ask yourself to consider the following questions:

- What situations or events tend to trigger stress in my life?
- How do I typically react to stress? Are there physical or emotional symptoms that accompany it?
- Are there recurring patterns or themes in the stressors I face?

2. Stress Journal:

Suggestions, keep a stress journal for a specified period (e.g., a week or a month). In your journal, record the following details whenever you experience stress:

- Date and time of the stressful event.
- Description of the event or situation that caused stress.
- Emotional reactions and feelings during and after the event.
- Physical symptoms experienced (e.g., headaches, muscle tension, racing heart).
- Any coping strategies or actions taken to deal with the stress.

By maintaining a stress journal, you can identify patterns and common triggers for your stress. This process can be eye-opening and help you gain insights into your stressors.

3. Self-Assessment Tools:

The use of self-assessment tools or questionnaires designed to pinpoint specific stressors in different areas of life. There are numerous stress assessment surveys available online or in self-help books that can help individuals identify sources of stress related to work, relationships, finances, and more. Encourage yourself to complete these assessments to gain a clearer picture of your stressors.

4. Seek Feedback:

Reach out to trusted friends, family members, or colleagues for feedback. Sometimes, others can offer valuable insights into our behavior and stressors that we might not be aware of. Prioritize in open and honest conversations where you can ask for input on areas of your life that may contribute to stress.

5. Professional Guidance:

If you find it challenging to identify your stressors or suspect that your stress is linked to deeper emotional or psychological issues, Its important you seeking professional guidance.

A mental health counsellor, therapist, or psychologist can provide valuable insights and tools for recognizing and addressing stressors.

6. Mindfulness and Mindful Observation:

Promote mindfulness practices. You can practice mindfulness by being fully present in others daily activities. Mindful observation can help them become more aware of their thoughts, emotions, and physical sensations in the moment. This heightened awareness can reveal stress triggers and patterns.

7. Gradual Exploration:

Remind yourself that recognizing stressors may not happen overnight. It's a gradual process that requires patienc

e and self-compassion. They may uncover stressors one by one, and that's perfectly normal. The key is to start the journey toward self-awareness.

By guiding yourself through these strategies, you can empower yourself to become more attuned to your stressors. Once you identify these sources of stress, you can then move on to the next steps of managing and mitigating their effectively, as explored in subsequent chapters.

Here are some exercises and worksheets that you can use for self-assessment to help them identify their sources of stress:

Exercise 1: Stress Journal

Purpose: This exercise involves keeping a stress journal to track and analyze stressors over a specific period.

Instructions:

1. Obtain a notebook or create a digital document to serve as your stress journal.
2. Set a specific duration for your journaling, such as a week or a month.
3. Each day, record the following information:
   - Date and time of the stressful event.
   - A brief description of the event or situation that caused stress.
   - Your emotional reactions and feelings during and after the event.
   - Any physical symptoms experienced (e.g., headaches, muscle tension, upset stomach).
   - Any coping strategies or actions you took to deal with the stress.
4. At the end of the designated period, review your journal entries and look for patterns or common stressors. Pay attention to situations, people, or circumstances that repeatedly appear.

Worksheet 1: Stress Assessment

Purpose: This worksheet is designed to help individuals assess stress in different areas of their life, such as work, relationships, and personal habits.

Instructions:

1. Create a table with three columns: "Area of Life," "Stressors," and "Impact on Well-being."
2. In the "Area of Life" column, list the various aspects of your life, such as work, family, relationships, health, finances, and personal habits.
3. In the "Stressors" column, write down specific stressors within each area. For example:
   - Area of Life: Work
     - Stressors: Heavy workload, tight deadlines, difficult coworkers.
   - Area of Life: Relationships
     - Stressors: Conflict with spouse, strained relationship with parents.
4. In the "Impact on Well-being" column, assess how each stressor affects your overall well-being on a scale of 1 to 10, with 1 being minimal impact and 10 being severe impact.
5. After completing the table, review your assessment to identify which areas of your life are most affected by stress and which specific stressors have the greatest impact.

Exercise 2: Mindful Observation

Purpose: Mindful observation is a mindfulness practice that helps individuals become more aware of their thoughts, emotions, and physical sensations, allowing them to recognize stress triggers.

Instructions:

1. Find a quiet and comfortable place to sit or lie down.
2. Close your eyes and take a few deep breaths to center yourself.
3. Begin to observe your thoughts without judgment. Notice any thoughts or worries that come to mind. Acknowledge them without trying to change or control them.
4. Shift your attention to your emotions. What emotions are you currently experiencing? Are there any emotions that stand out as particularly strong?
5. Gradually bring your awareness to your physical sensations. Pay attention to any areas of tension or discomfort in your body. Are there any physical signs of stress, such as muscle tension or a racing heart?

6. Spend at least 5-10 minutes in mindful observation, simply being present and aware of your inner experiences.
7. Afterward, reflect on any thoughts, emotions, or physical sensations that arose during the practice. Are there recurring themes or triggers that you notice?

These exercises and worksheets can help readers gain valuable insights into their sources of stress. By consistently practicing self-assessment and mindfulness, individuals can become more attuned to their stressors and take proactive steps to address them effectively.

Encouraging Mindfulness and Self-Awareness

Mindfulness and self-awareness are powerful tools for managing stress and improving overall well-being. By promoting these practices, you can empower readers to become more attuned to their thoughts, emotions, and physical sensations, helping them identify and navigate their sources of stress effectively. Here are some tips and exercises to encourage mindfulness and self-awareness:

1. Mindfulness Meditation:

- **Guided Meditation:** Encourage readers to try guided mindfulness meditation sessions available online or through mobile apps. These guided sessions can provide structured guidance for beginners.
- **Breathing Exercises:** Teach simple mindfulness breathing exercises, such as deep belly breathing. Instruct readers to focus on their breath and observe each inhalation and exhalation.

2. Mindful Observation:

- **Daily Routine:** Encourage readers to incorporate moments of mindful observation into their daily routine. For example, while eating a meal, they can Savor each bite, paying attention to taste, texture, and aroma.
- **Nature Walk:** Suggest taking a mindful nature walk where they observe the sights, sounds, and sensations of the natural environment. Encourage them to notice the details in leaves, the chirping of birds, and the feeling of the breeze.

3. Journaling:

- **Emotional Journaling:** Suggest keeping an emotional journal where readers record their feelings and emotional responses throughout the day. This practice can help them gain insights into patterns of stress and triggers.
- **Gratitude Journal:** Recommend maintaining a gratitude journal where readers jot down things they are thankful for daily. Focusing on gratitude can shift their perspective and reduce stress.

4. Body Scan:

- **Progressive Muscle Relaxation:** Guide readers through a body scan exercise where they systematically focus on each part of their body, releasing tension and promoting relaxation.

5. Mindful Breathing Techniques:

- **Box Breathing:** Teach the "box breathing" technique, where readers inhale for a count of four, hold for four, exhale for four, and pause for four before repeating. This practice can help regulate stress responses.

6. Self-Reflection:

- **Daily Self-Check:** Encourage readers to set aside a few minutes each day for self-reflection. They can ask themselves how they are feeling emotionally, physically, and mentally.

7. Mindful Eating:

- **Sensory Experience:** Encourage readers to practice mindful eating by savouring each bite, paying attention to flavours and textures. Discourage distractions like screens or multitasking during meals.

8. Mindful Listening:

- **Active Listening:** Suggest that readers practice active listening in their interactions with others. Encourage them to fully engage in conversations, giving their complete attention to the speaker.

9. Guided Mindfulness Apps:

- Recommend mindfulness and meditation apps that offer guided sessions, such as Headspace, Calm, or Insight Timer. These apps provide structured practices for building mindfulness skills.

10. Group Mindfulness:

- Encourage readers to explore group mindfulness activities, such as yoga classes, meditation groups, or mindfulness workshops in their community. Group settings can enhance the mindfulness experience.

Remind readers that mindfulness and self-awareness are skills that improve with practice and patience. By regularly incorporating these practices into their lives, they can develop a greater understanding of themselves, their stressors, and how to respond to challenges with greater resilience and calmness.

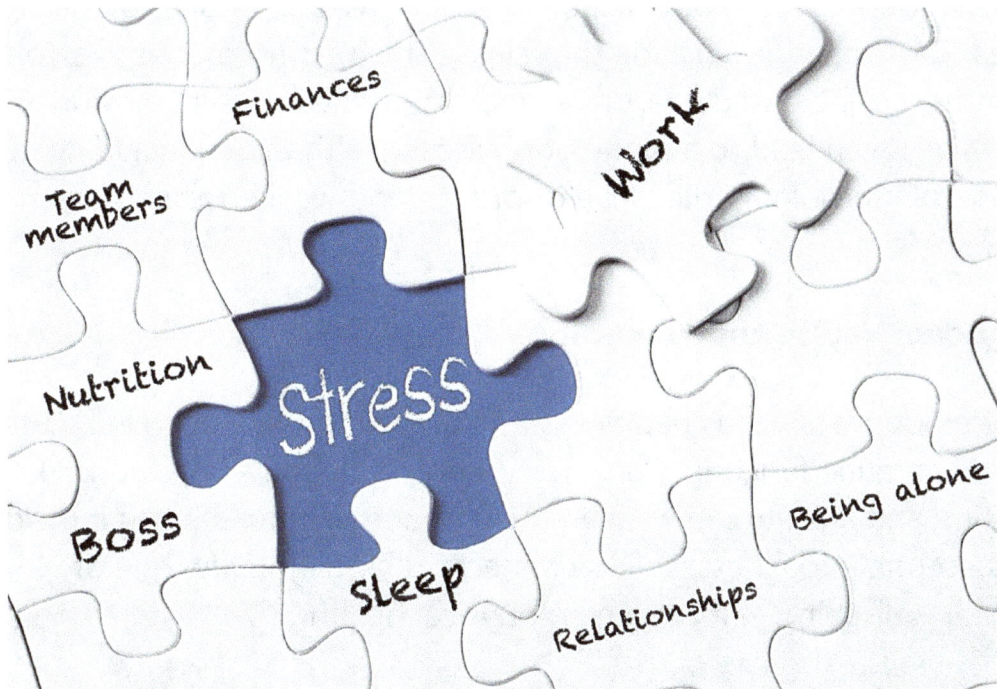

Fig. 2: Some of the notorious sources of stress

Chapter 3

Harmonizing Harmony: The Profound Influence of Your Mind on Your Body

The intricate interplay between the mind and the body is a fascinating and powerful aspect of our human experience. In this chapter, we will delve into the concept of the mind-body connection and explore how our mental and emotional well-being profoundly impacts our physical health.

Understanding the Mind-Body Connection:

The mind-body connection refers to the bidirectional relationship between our thoughts, emotions, beliefs, and our physical health. It's a dynamic interplay where our mental and emotional states can influence our physical well-being and vice versa. Here are some key aspects to consider:

1. Stress and Physical Health:

Stress serves as a prime example of the mind-body connection. When we experience stress, whether it's due to work pressure, relationship difficulties, or financial worries, our body responds with a cascade of physiological changes. These changes include the release of stress hormones like cortisol and adrenaline, increased heart rate, and heightened muscle tension. Chronic stress can lead to a range of physical health issues, including cardiovascular problems, digestive disorders, and weakened immune function.

2. Emotional Health and Immunity:

Positive emotions, such as happiness and gratitude, have been linked to improved immune function. Conversely, chronic negative emotions like depression and anxiety can weaken the immune system, making individuals more susceptible to illnesses. This connection highlights the role of emotional well-being in maintaining physical health.

3. Pain Perception:

The mind has a significant influence on how we perceive and experience pain. Studies have shown that factors like stress, anxiety, and negative thoughts can intensify the experience of pain, while relaxation techniques and positive distractions can alleviate it. This demonstrates the power of the mind in modulating physical sensations.

4. Placebo Effect:

The placebo effect is a phenomenon where individuals experience improvements in their symptoms or conditions after receiving a treatment with no active therapeutic ingredient. This effect underscores the mind's ability to influence physical outcomes, as belief in the treatment can lead to actual physiological changes.

Cultivating a Positive Mind-Body Connection:

Now that we understand the mind-body connection's significance, let's explore how readers can cultivate a positive and harmonious relationship between their mental and physical well-being:

1. Mindful Awareness:

Encourage readers to practice mindfulness to become more aware of their thoughts, emotions, and physical sensations. Mindfulness can help them recognize stressors and negative thought patterns, allowing for conscious choices to mitigate their impact.

2. Stress Reduction Techniques:

Teach stress reduction techniques such as meditation, deep breathing exercises, and progressive muscle relaxation. These practices can help individuals manage stress effectively, preventing its adverse effects on physical health.

3. Emotional Expression:

Promote healthy emotional expression. Encourage readers to express their emotions constructively rather than suppressing them. Emotional release can prevent the buildup of emotional stress that negatively affects the body.

4. Positive Visualization:

Guide readers to use the power of positive visualization. Help them visualize desired physical outcomes and believe in the body's capacity to heal and thrive. Positive thoughts and expectations can have a profound impact on recovery and well-being.

5. Physical Activity:

Highlight the importance of regular physical activity for both mental and physical health. Exercise releases endorphins, which are natural mood lifters, and helps reduce stress.

6. Balanced Lifestyle:

Emphasize the need for a balanced lifestyle that includes adequate sleep, a healthy diet, and regular relaxation. These factors contribute to both mental and physical well-being.

7. Seek Professional Help:

Encourage readers to seek professional guidance when dealing with chronic stress, mental health issues, or physical conditions. Therapists, counsellors, and medical professionals can provide valuable support and treatment.

In this chapter, readers will explore the profound ways in which their mental and emotional states influence their physical health. By understanding and nurturing the mind-body connection, individuals can take proactive steps to promote holistic well-being and embark on a path towards a healthier, more balanced life.

Exploring the Connection Between Mental and Physical Health

The connection between mental and physical health is a complex and intricate one, with each aspect of well-being profoundly influencing the other. This mind-body interaction highlights how our thoughts, emotions, and behaviours impact our physical health, and vice versa. Here's a closer look at the key elements of this connection:

1. Stress and Its Physical Toll:

Stress is a prime example of how mental and emotional states can affect physical health. When we experience stress, whether due to work pressures, relationship difficulties, or other factors, our body responds with a series of physiological changes. These changes include increased heart rate, elevated blood pressure, and the release of stress hormones like cortisol and adrenaline.

Chronic stress can lead to a range of physical health problems, including:

- **Cardiovascular Issues:** Prolonged stress is linked to heart disease, hypertension, and an increased risk of heart attacks and strokes.
- **Digestive Disorders:** Stress can disrupt normal digestive processes, leading to conditions like irritable bowel syndrome (IBS) and indigestion.
- **Weakened Immune Function:** Stress weakens the immune system, making the body more susceptible to infections and illnesses.

2. The Immune System and Emotional Well-Being:

The immune system plays a crucial role in defending the body against illness. Studies have shown that emotions and mental states can influence immune function. For example:

- **Positive Emotions:** Feelings of happiness, gratitude, and optimism are associated with improved immune function. Positive emotions can enhance the body's ability to fight off infections and illnesses.
- **Negative Emotions:** Chronic negative emotions, such as depression and anxiety, can weaken the immune system, increasing vulnerability to illnesses.

3. Pain Perception and Mental State:

The mind has a significant influence on how individuals perceive and experience pain. Factors such as stress, anxiety, and negative thoughts can intensify the experience of pain. Conversely, relaxation techniques, positive distractions, and a positive mental outlook can alleviate pain.

4. Lifestyle Behaviours:

Mental and emotional states can influence lifestyle choices that impact physical health. For example:

- **Depression:** Individuals with depression may be more prone to unhealthy behaviours like overeating, leading to weight gain and related health issues.
- **Stress:** Chronic stress can lead to coping behaviours such as smoking, excessive alcohol consumption, or unhealthy eating habits.

5. The Placebo Effect:

The placebo effect demonstrates the mind's power to influence physical outcomes. When individuals believe they are receiving a treatment, even if it has no active therapeutic ingredient, they may experience real physiological changes and symptom improvements. This phenomenon underscores the role of belief and expectation in healing and recovery.

6. Chronic Conditions and Mental Health:

Managing chronic physical conditions, such as diabetes, heart disease, or chronic pain, often requires a holistic approach that addresses mental and emotional well-being. Mental health issues like depression or anxiety can complicate the management of chronic conditions and affect treatment adherence.

7. The Role of Coping Mechanisms:

How individuals cope with stress and adversity can significantly impact both their mental and physical health. Healthy coping mechanisms, such as exercise, mindfulness, and seeking social support, can improve mental well-being and have positive effects on physical health.

Understanding the profound connection between mental and physical health underscores the importance of holistic well-being. Nurturing both mental and physical health through stress management, emotional well-being, and healthy lifestyle choices is essential for achieving a balanced and vibrant life. Recognizing this connection empowers individuals to take proactive steps to enhance their overall well-being and resilience in the face of life's challenges.

The Role of Stress in Chronic Illnesses

Stress is a significant contributor to the development and exacerbation of chronic illnesses. The relationship between chronic conditions and stress is complex, involving both physiological and behavioural factors. Here's an exploration of the role of stress in chronic illnesses:

1. Stress as a Trigger:

Stress can serve as a trigger for the onset of chronic illnesses, particularly in individuals who are genetically predisposed to these conditions. Stress activates the body's "fight or flight" response, leading to physiological changes that can be harmful when chronically activated. This includes increased heart rate, elevated blood pressure, and the release of stress hormones like cortisol. Over time, these responses can contribute to the development of chronic conditions.

2. Impact on Cardiovascular Health:

Chronic stress is closely linked to cardiovascular diseases, including:

- **Hypertension (High Blood Pressure):** Prolonged stress can lead to persistently elevated blood pressure, which is a significant risk factor for heart disease and stroke.
- **Coronary Heart Disease:** Stress can contribute to the buildup of plaque in the arteries, increasing the risk of coronary heart disease, heart attacks, and angina.
- **Arrhythmias:** Stress can trigger abnormal heart rhythms, which can be harmful for individuals with underlying heart conditions.

3. Immune System Suppression:

Stress weakens the immune system, making the body more susceptible to infections and illnesses. Chronic stress can lead to immune system dysfunction, increasing the risk of infections, autoimmune disorders, and slower healing from injuries or surgeries.

4. Inflammation and Chronic Conditions:

Stress can contribute to chronic inflammation in the body, which is a common factor in many chronic illnesses, including:

- **Type 2 Diabetes:** Chronic inflammation can lead to insulin resistance and impair blood sugar regulation, contributing to the development of diabetes.
- **Autoimmune Diseases:** Stress may exacerbate autoimmune conditions like rheumatoid arthritis, lupus, and multiple sclerosis by promoting inflammation and immune system dysfunction.

5. Mental Health and Chronic Illness:

The relationship between chronic illness and mental health is bidirectional. Chronic illnesses can lead to stress, anxiety, and depression due to the challenges of managing the condition and the impact on quality of life. Conversely, the psychological distress associated with chronic conditions can exacerbate symptoms and impair overall well-being.

6. Unhealthy Coping Behaviours:

When individuals experience chronic stress, they may turn to unhealthy coping mechanisms such as smoking, excessive alcohol consumption, overeating, or drug use. These behaviours can further contribute to the development of chronic illnesses, including respiratory conditions, heart disease, and obesity.

7. Impact on Lifestyle:

Stress can disrupt healthy lifestyle habits, such as regular exercise, balanced nutrition, and adequate sleep. These disruptions can contribute to chronic illnesses like obesity, metabolic syndrome, and sleep disorders.

8. Exacerbation of Pre-existing Conditions:

For individuals with pre-existing chronic conditions, stress can exacerbate symptoms and lead to disease progression. Stress-induced inflammation and hormonal changes can worsen the course of conditions such as irritable bowel syndrome (IBS), migraine, and chronic pain syndromes.

Recognizing the role of stress in chronic illnesses highlights the importance of stress management as a critical component of preventive healthcare and disease management. Implementing stress reduction techniques, seeking social support, and addressing mental health concerns can help individuals reduce their susceptibility to chronic illnesses and improve their overall quality of life. Additionally, healthcare professionals often consider stress management strategies as part of the treatment plan for individuals with chronic conditions to optimize their health outcomes.

Introduction to Relaxation Techniques and Their Benefits

In today's fast-paced and often stressful world, relaxation techniques offer a powerful antidote to the demands and pressures of daily life. These techniques are valuable tools for achieving a state of mental and physical calm, reducing stress, and promoting overall well-being. In this section, we'll introduce various relaxation techniques and explore their numerous benefits:

What Are Relaxation Techniques?

Relaxation techniques encompass a wide range of practices and exercises designed to induce a state of relaxation and ease tension in both the mind and body. These techniques are grounded in the principles of mindfulness, breath control, and the release of physical tension.

Types of Relaxation Techniques:

There are several well-established relaxation techniques, each with its own unique approach to achieving relaxation:

1. **Deep Breathing:** Deep breathing exercises involve slow, intentional breaths that engage the diaphragm. This technique helps reduce stress by calming the body's "fight or flight" response and promoting relaxation.
2. **Progressive Muscle Relaxation:** This practice involves systematically tensing and then relaxing different muscle groups to release physical tension. It's effective for relieving muscle stiffness and reducing stress.

3. **Meditation:** Meditation is a mindfulness practice that involves focusing one's attention and eliminating the stream of jumbled thoughts that crowd the mind. It cultivates mental clarity, emotional balance, and relaxation.
4. **Yoga:** Yoga combines physical postures, breath control, and mindfulness to promote relaxation, flexibility, and stress reduction. It also enhances physical strength and balance.
5. **Tai Chi:** Tai Chi is a mind-body practice characterized by slow, flowing movements and deep breathing. It enhances relaxation, balance, and overall physical and mental well-being.
6. **Visualization:** Visualization techniques involve imagining peaceful and calming scenes or situations. This practice can reduce stress and anxiety by shifting focus away from sources of tension.
7. **Autogenic Training:** This relaxation method involves using verbal cues and imagery to promote relaxation by focusing on bodily sensations and promoting self-regulation.

Benefits of Relaxation Techniques:

The benefits of incorporating relaxation techniques into your daily life are numerous and profound:

1. **Stress Reduction:** Relaxation techniques are highly effective in reducing stress levels, helping individuals better manage the challenges of everyday life.
2. **Improved Mental Health:** Regular practice of relaxation techniques can alleviate symptoms of anxiety, depression, and other mental health disorders. It promotes emotional balance and resilience.
3. **Better Sleep:** Relaxation promotes better sleep by calming the mind and reducing insomnia and sleep disturbances.
4. **Pain Management:** Techniques like progressive muscle relaxation and mindfulness can help manage chronic pain conditions by reducing muscle tension and altering pain perception.
5. **Enhanced Focus and Concentration:** Relaxation techniques improve concentration and cognitive function by reducing mental clutter and promoting mental clarity.

6. **Strengthened Immune System:** Reduced stress and improved overall well-being support a stronger immune system, reducing susceptibility to illness.
7. **Lower Blood Pressure:** Deep breathing exercises and relaxation practices can help lower blood pressure, reducing the risk of cardiovascular diseases.
8. **Enhanced Physical Health:** Yoga and Tai Chi, in particular, enhance physical health by promoting flexibility, strength, and balance.
9. **Improved Quality of Life:** Ultimately, relaxation techniques contribute to an improved quality of life by fostering a sense of inner peace, balance, and well-being.

As we delve deeper into the various relaxation techniques in the following chapters, you will discover practical guidance on how to incorporate these practices into your daily routine. Whether you are seeking stress relief, improved mental health, or physical well-being, relaxation techniques offer a path to greater calm and vitality in your life.

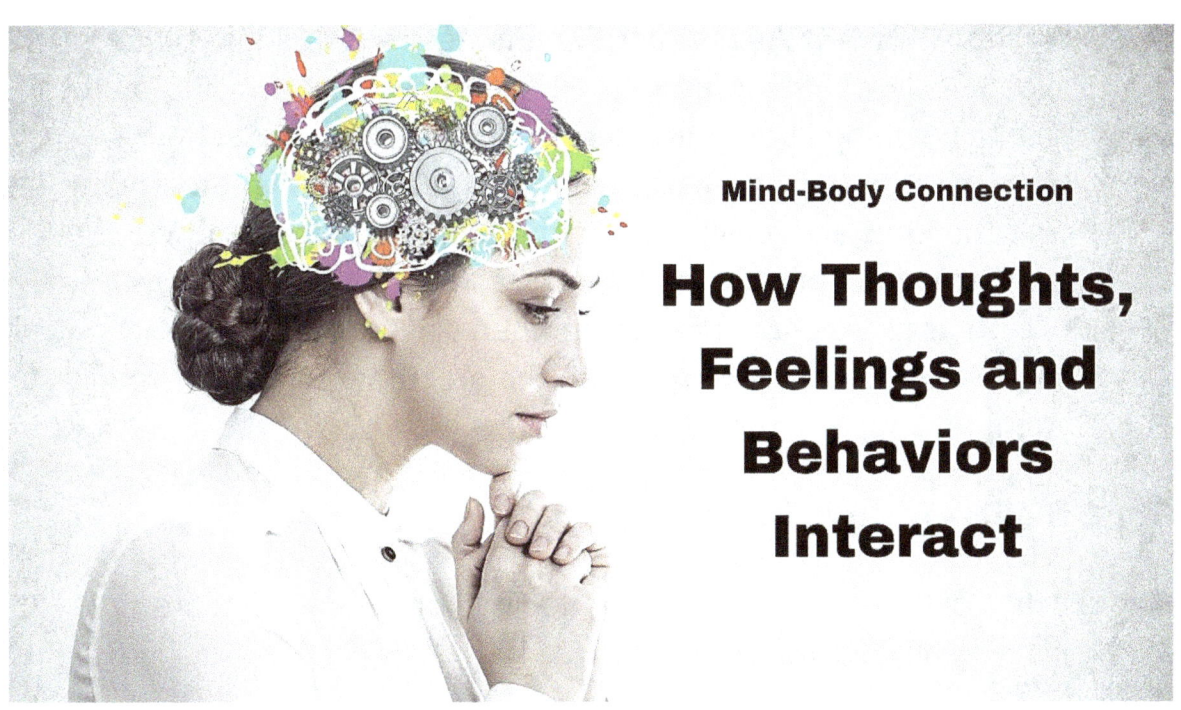

Chapter 4

Awakening the Present Moment: Harnessing Mindfulness for a Stress-Free Life

Mindfulness, a practice rooted in ancient traditions, has gained recognition in recent years as a potent tool for reducing stress and enhancing overall well-being. In this chapter, we explore the transformative power of mindfulness and its role in cultivating a stress-free life.

Understanding Mindfulness:

Mindfulness is the art of being fully present in the moment, without judgment or distraction. It involves paying deliberate attention to your thoughts, emotions, bodily sensations, and the world around you. At its core, mindfulness is about observing your inner and outer experiences with a curious, non-reactive awareness.

Key Principles of Mindfulness:

1. **Present-Moment Awareness:** Mindfulness encourages you to engage fully with the present moment, rather than dwelling on the past or worrying about the future.
2. **Non-Judgmental Acceptance:** Mindfulness invites you to accept your thoughts and feelings without judgment. It encourages a compassionate attitude toward yourself and your experiences.
3. **Breath as an Anchor:** The breath often serves as an anchor in mindfulness practice. Focusing on the breath helps ground your attention and calm the mind.

The Benefits of Mindfulness:

The practice of mindfulness offers a wide array of benefits that are particularly relevant to living a stress-free life:

1. **Stress Reduction:** Mindfulness has been shown to reduce stress by helping individuals manage their reactions to stressors and promoting relaxation.
2. **Emotional Regulation:** Mindfulness enhances emotional regulation by increasing awareness of emotions and providing tools for responding to them skilfully.

3. **Improved Concentration:** Regular mindfulness practice enhances focus and concentration, making it easier to complete tasks and stay present in daily activities.
4. **Enhanced Well-Being:** Mindfulness contributes to greater overall well-being, fostering positive emotions, gratitude, and contentment.
5. **Better Sleep:** Mindfulness techniques promote relaxation and reduce racing thoughts, leading to improved sleep quality.
6. **Pain Management:** Mindfulness can be an effective tool for managing chronic pain by changing the perception of pain and reducing muscle tension.

Incorporating Mindfulness into Daily Life:

This chapter will provide practical guidance on incorporating mindfulness into your daily routine. Some strategies include:

1. **Mindful Breathing:** Learn breathing exercises that serve as a foundation for mindfulness. These exercises can be practiced anywhere, anytime.
2. **Meditation:** Explore mindfulness meditation practices, ranging from short, guided sessions to longer, self-guided ones.
3. **Mindful Eating:** Discover how to bring mindfulness to your eating habits, savouring each bite and cultivating a healthier relationship with food.
4. **Mindful Movement:** Explore mindfulness in motion through practices like walking meditation and mindful yoga.
5. **Mindful Living:** Learn how to apply mindfulness to everyday activities, such as driving, working, and communicating with others.

Cultivating a Stress-Free Life with Mindfulness:

As you delve into the practice of mindfulness, you'll uncover the profound influence it can have on your ability to navigate life's challenges with grace and resilience. By embracing mindfulness, you will awaken to the richness of each moment and gain powerful tools for living a life free from the grip of stress. This chapter is your gateway to unlocking the transformative potential of mindfulness and harnessing it for your own well-being.

Defining Mindfulness and Its Role in Stress Reduction

Mindfulness is a mental practice that involves paying deliberate and non-judgmental attention to the present moment. It's about being fully aware of your thoughts, emotions, bodily sensations, and the environment around you without trying to change or judge them. Mindfulness cultivates a state of focused, open, and accepting awareness.

The Role of Mindfulness in Stress Reduction:

Mindfulness plays a pivotal role in stress reduction and management by changing how individuals perceive and respond to stressors. Here's how mindfulness contributes to a stress-free life:

1. **Awareness of Stress Triggers:** Mindfulness helps individuals become more attuned to their stressors. By being present and mindful, you can recognize the early signs of stress as they arise, allowing you to address them proactively.
2. **Reduced Reactivity:** Mindfulness fosters a non-reactive attitude. Instead of automatically reacting to stress with tension or anxiety, individuals learn to observe their responses without judgment. This non-reactivity reduces the emotional intensity of stress.
3. **Improved Emotional Regulation:** Mindfulness enhances emotional regulation by promoting a balanced response to emotions. It allows individuals to acknowledge and validate their feelings while preventing them from overwhelming or controlling their actions.
4. **Enhanced Coping Strategies:** Mindfulness equips individuals with effective coping strategies for managing stress. Techniques such as deep breathing and meditation provide tools for calming the nervous system and reducing stress-related symptoms.
5. **Increased Resilience:** Regular mindfulness practice strengthens resilience—the ability to bounce back from stress and adversity. Mindfulness teaches individuals to adapt to challenges with greater ease and flexibility.
6. **Stress Reduction through Relaxation:** Mindfulness practices, such as mindful breathing and progressive muscle relaxation, induce a relaxation response in the body. This counteracts the physiological effects of stress, reducing muscle tension, lowering blood pressure, and promoting overall relaxation.

7. **Enhanced Focus and Clarity:** Mindfulness improves cognitive function, including focus and concentration. This allows individuals to approach tasks and problem-solving with a clear mind, reducing the sense of overwhelm associated with stress.

8. **Mindful Coping with Uncertainty:** Mindfulness helps individuals cope with uncertainty and uncontrollable aspects of life. By accepting the present moment as it is, individuals can reduce the anxiety and stress associated with trying to control the uncontrollable.

9. **Improved Sleep:** Mindfulness techniques can alleviate insomnia and sleep disturbances by calming the mind and reducing racing thoughts that often interfere with sleep.

10. **Positive Outlook:** Mindfulness fosters a positive outlook on life. By training the mind to focus on the present moment and cultivate gratitude, individuals can reduce negative rumination and increase feelings of contentment.

Overall, mindfulness promotes a state of balance and calm, allowing individuals to respond to life's challenges with greater equanimity. It shifts the focus from dwelling on the past or worrying about the future to fully experiencing and appreciating the richness of the present moment. By integrating mindfulness into their daily lives, individuals can significantly reduce stress and enhance their overall well-being.

Certainly! Here are some practical mindfulness exercises and tips to help you incorporate mindfulness into your daily life:

1. Mindful Breathing:

- **Exercise:** Find a quiet space, sit comfortably, and close your eyes. Take a deep breath in through your nose for a count of four, hold for four, and then exhale slowly through your mouth for four. Focus your attention on the sensation of your breath. Repeat this for a few minutes.
- **Tip:** Practice mindful breathing when you're feeling stressed or overwhelmed. It's a quick way to centre yourself and calm your mind.

2. Body Scan:

- **Exercise:** Lie down or sit in a comfortable position. Start at the top of your head and slowly scan your body, paying attention to any areas of tension or discomfort. As you identify these areas, consciously relax and release the tension.
- **Tip:** Use the body scan to relax before bedtime or when you're feeling physically tense.

3. Mindful Eating:

- **Exercise:** During a meal, eat slowly and savour each bite. Pay attention to the taste, texture, and aroma of your food. Put down your utensils between bites and engage all your senses in the eating experience.
- **Tip:** Practice mindful eating to prevent overeating and develop a healthier relationship with food.

4. Five Senses Exercise:

- **Exercise:** Pause and identify:
  - Five things you can see.
  - Four things you can touch.
  - Three things you can hear.
  - Two things you can smell.
  - One thing you can taste.
- **Tip:** Use this exercise to ground yourself in the present moment, especially when you're feeling anxious or distracted.

5. Mindful Walking:

- **Exercise:** Take a slow, mindful walk. Pay attention to the sensation of each step, the feeling of the ground beneath your feet, and the rhythm of your breath. Notice the sights and sounds around you without judgment.
- **Tip:** Incorporate mindful walking into your daily routine, such as during a lunch break or when walking your dog.

6. Gratitude Journal:

- **Exercise:** Dedicate a few minutes each day to write down three things you're grateful for. Reflect on why you're thankful for these things.
- **Tip:** Practicing gratitude can shift your focus from stressors to positive aspects of your life.

7. Mindful Communication:

- **Exercise:** In conversations, practice active listening. Give your full attention to the speaker without planning your response. Listen empathetically and without judgment.
- **Tip:** Mindful communication can improve relationships and reduce misunderstandings.

8. Mindful Technology Use:

- **Exercise:** Set aside specific times to check emails, social media, or news updates. When using technology, do so intentionally and avoid mindless scrolling or multitasking.
- **Tip:** Mindful technology use can help reduce information overload and screen-related stress.

9. Mindful Moments:

- **Exercise:** Incorporate short moments of mindfulness throughout your day. Pause for a minute to take a few mindful breaths, even during routine tasks like washing dishes or waiting in line.
- **Tip:** These micro-moments of mindfulness can add up and make a significant difference in your stress levels.

10. Guided Meditation:

- **Exercise:** Find guided mindfulness meditation sessions or apps led by experienced instructors. Follow along with these guided sessions, which can range from a few minutes to longer practices.
- **Tip:** Guided meditations provide structure and guidance, making it easier to establish a regular mindfulness practice.

Remember that mindfulness is a skill that develops with practice. Start with shorter sessions and gradually extend the duration as you become more comfortable. Consistency is key, so aim to integrate mindfulness into your daily routine to experience its full benefits in stress reduction and overall well-being.

Here are a couple of real-life success stories that highlight the transformative power of mindfulness in reducing stress and improving overall well-being:

1. Jon Kabat-Zinn and the Mindfulness-Based Stress Reduction (MBSR) Program:

Jon Kabat-Zinn is a pioneer in bringing mindfulness to mainstream healthcare. In the late 1970s, Kabat-Zinn, a molecular biologist and meditation practitioner, developed the Mindfulness-Based Stress Reduction (MBSR) program at the University of Massachusetts Medical School. The program aimed to help individuals with chronic pain and stress-related conditions.

Success Story: One of the early participants in the MBSR program was a woman named Mary, who had been struggling with chronic back pain and severe stress due to her demanding job. After completing the program, Mary reported significant reductions in her pain levels and a newfound ability to cope with stress. She found that mindfulness not only improved her physical health but also enhanced her overall quality of life. Inspired by her experience, Mary went on to become an MBSR instructor, helping countless others find relief from chronic conditions and stress.

2. Corporations Embracing Mindfulness:

Numerous corporations and organizations have introduced mindfulness programs for their employees to enhance well-being and productivity. Google is a prominent example of a company that has embraced mindfulness.

Success Story: Chade-Meng Tan, a former Google engineer, initiated the "Search Inside Yourself" program at Google in 2007, which introduced mindfulness and emotional intelligence training to employees. The program was met with remarkable success. Employees reported reduced stress levels, improved focus, and greater job satisfaction. As the program expanded, it influenced the company's culture, fostering a more compassionate and mindful work environment. Other organizations, such as Adobe and General Mills, have also implemented mindfulness programs with similar positive outcomes, demonstrating how mindfulness can benefit both employees and the workplace as a whole.

These success stories illustrate how mindfulness can be a catalyst for profound positive change in individuals' lives, from managing chronic pain and stress to creating more mindful and compassionate work environments. They serve as inspiring examples of the potential for mindfulness to improve well-being and enhance the quality of life in various settings and contexts.

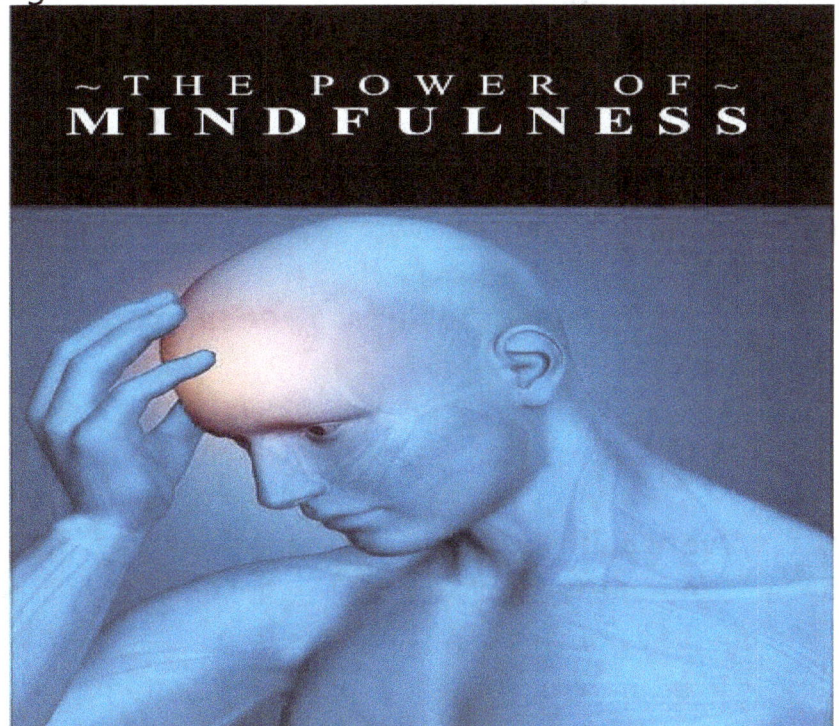

Chapter 5

Time Management and Prioritization

Mastering the Clock: Strategies for a Stress-Free Life through Effective Time Management

In the quest for a stress-free life, time management and prioritization are indispensable tools. In this chapter, we explore the art and science of managing your time wisely to reduce stress, increase productivity, and achieve a sense of balance and fulfillment.

Understanding Time Management:

Time management is the process of planning and organizing your tasks and activities to make the most efficient use of your time. It involves setting goals, prioritizing responsibilities, and allocating your resources effectively to accomplish what matters most to you.

The Role of Time Management in Stress Reduction:

Effective time management plays a pivotal role in reducing stress. Here's how it contributes to a stress-free life:

1. **Reduces Overwhelm:** When you manage your time well, you can break tasks into manageable chunks, reducing the feeling of being overwhelmed by numerous responsibilities.
2. **Enhances Productivity:** Time management strategies help you work more efficiently, allowing you to accomplish tasks in less time and with less effort.
3. **Creates Space for Relaxation:** By prioritizing and allocating time for relaxation and self-care, you ensure that you have moments of respite from the demands of daily life.

4. **Prevents Procrastination:** Effective time management strategies can help you overcome procrastination, reducing the stress that can arise from putting off important tasks.
5. **Improves Work-Life Balance:** When you allocate time for both work and personal life, you create a healthier work-life balance, reducing the stress associated with burnout and neglecting personal needs.

Practical Time Management Tips:

1. **Set Clear Goals:** Start with clear, achievable goals that align with your values and priorities. Knowing what you want to accomplish will guide your time management decisions.
2. **Prioritize Tasks:** Use techniques like the Eisenhower Matrix (urgent/important grid) to categorize tasks into four quadrants: urgent and important, not urgent but important, urgent but not important, and neither urgent nor important. Focus on the important tasks.
3. **Create a To-Do List:** Each day, create a to-do list with tasks ranked by priority. Tackle the most important tasks first, and avoid overloading your list.
4. **Time Blocking:** Allocate specific blocks of time for different tasks or activities. This helps prevent multitasking and ensures focused work.
5. **Eliminate Distractions:** Identify and eliminate common distractions like social media, excessive notifications, or a cluttered workspace that can derail your productivity.
6. **Set Boundaries:** Establish boundaries by communicating your work hours and availability to colleagues, family, and friends to protect your personal time.
7. **Learn to Say No:** Be selective about accepting additional commitments. Saying no when necessary is crucial for managing your time effectively.
8. **Delegate When Possible:** Delegate tasks that others can handle, whether at work or home. Delegation frees up your time for more critical responsibilities.
9. **Time Audit:** Periodically conduct a time audit to assess how you're spending your time. Identify areas where you can make improvements.

10. **Self-Care Time:** Schedule regular self-care activities, such as exercise, meditation, or hobbies, to recharge and reduce stress.

Technology and Time Management:

Utilize technology tools, such as calendar apps, task management apps, and productivity software, to streamline your time management efforts. These tools can help you stay organized, set reminders, and track your progress toward your goals.

Balancing Work and Personal Life:

Striking a balance between work and personal life is essential for a stress-free life. This chapter will also provide strategies for achieving a healthy work-life balance, including setting boundaries, managing work-related stress, and nurturing personal relationships.

In mastering the art of time management and prioritization, you'll equip yourself with invaluable skills for reducing stress, achieving your goals, and living a more balanced and fulfilling life.

The Importance of Time Management in Stress Reduction

Time management is a foundational skill for reducing stress and achieving a more balanced and fulfilling life. Here's a detailed exploration of why effective time management is crucial in stress reduction:

1. Prioritization of Responsibilities:

Time management involves identifying and prioritizing tasks and responsibilities. By differentiating between what is urgent and what is important, you can allocate your time and energy to tasks that truly matter. This prioritization prevents the feeling of being overwhelmed by a never-ending to-do list and reduces stress associated with the fear of not completing essential tasks.

2. Increased Efficiency:

Efficient time management techniques, such as setting clear goals, using to-do lists, and time blocking, enable you to work more effectively. You can complete tasks in less time and with less effort. This efficiency reduces the stress that arises from feeling constantly rushed and pressured to meet deadlines.

3. Prevention of Procrastination:

Procrastination is a common source of stress. When tasks are continually delayed, they accumulate and become more daunting, leading to increased anxiety and stress. Effective time management strategies help you overcome procrastination by breaking tasks into manageable steps and setting specific deadlines.

4. Creation of Time for Relaxation:

One of the fundamental principles of stress reduction is the inclusion of relaxation and self-care in your daily routine. Time management allows you to allocate time for relaxation and hobbies. This dedicated "me time" is essential for recharging, reducing stress, and preventing burnout.

5. Improved Work-Life Balance:

A healthy work-life balance is vital for well-being. Effective time management ensures that you allocate sufficient time to both professional and personal aspects of your life. This balance reduces the stress that can result from overcommitting to work and neglecting personal needs and relationships.

6. Reduced Overwhelm:

When you organize your tasks and responsibilities effectively, you can avoid the feeling of being overwhelmed. Knowing what needs to be done and having a plan to tackle it instils a sense of control and confidence, reducing stress related to uncertainty and chaos.

7. Enhanced Focus and Productivity:

Time management techniques encourage focused work. When you allocate specific blocks of time to tasks and eliminate distractions, you can work with heightened concentration. Improved focus and productivity reduce stress caused by feelings of ineffectiveness and inadequacy.

8. Better Stress Coping Mechanisms:

Effective time management promotes resilience in the face of stress. By managing your time wisely, you create opportunities to engage in stress-reduction practices such as exercise, mindfulness, and relaxation. These coping mechanisms become integral to your routine, helping you better manage and mitigate stress.

9. Goal Achievement and Fulfillment:

Time management enables you to set and pursue your goals effectively. When you make progress toward your goals, you experience a sense of accomplishment and fulfillment. This positive feedback loop reduces stress by increasing your sense of purpose and satisfaction.

10. Improved Decision-Making:

Time management encourages thoughtful decision-making. You have the time and mental clarity to make informed choices about your commitments and priorities. Avoiding impulsive or reactive decisions reduces stress caused by overcommitment and regret.

In essence, effective time management is a cornerstone of stress reduction. It empowers you to take control of your time, allocate it wisely, and create a balanced and fulfilling life. By mastering time management techniques, you equip yourself with valuable tools for reducing stress, increasing productivity, and achieving a greater sense of well-being and resilience.

Certainly! Effective time management involves using tools and strategies to make the most of your time and achieve your goals while reducing stress. Here are some valuable tools and strategies to help you manage your time effectively:

Time Management Tools:

1. **Calendar Apps:** Use digital calendar apps like Google Calendar, Apple Calendar, or Microsoft Outlook to schedule appointments, set deadlines, and receive reminders.
2. **Task Management Apps:** Task management apps like Todoist, Trello, or Asana help you create to-do lists, set priorities, and track progress on tasks and projects.
3. **Time Tracking Software:** Tools like Toggl or Clockify help you monitor how you spend your time. Tracking your activities can reveal areas where you can improve efficiency.
4. **Note-Taking Apps:** Apps like Evernote or OneNote are helpful for jotting down ideas, goals, and tasks. You can organize and access your notes easily.
5. **Project Management Software:** For complex projects, consider using project management software such as Monday.com or Basecamp to plan, allocate resources, and track progress.
6. **Pomodoro Timer Apps:** The Pomodoro Technique involves working in focused 25-minute intervals (Pomodoros) with short breaks in between. Apps like Focus Booster or Pomodone can help implement this technique.

Time Management Strategies:

1. **Set Clear Goals:** Define your short-term and long-term goals. Having clear objectives gives your tasks purpose and helps you prioritize effectively.
2. **Prioritize Tasks:** Use the Eisenhower Matrix (urgent/important grid) to categorize tasks as urgent and important, not urgent but important, urgent but not important, or neither urgent nor important. Focus on the important tasks.
3. **Create a To-Do List:** Daily to-do lists keep you organized and provide a visual representation of your tasks. Prioritize items on your list to tackle the most important ones first.

4. **Time Blocking:** Allocate specific time blocks for different tasks or categories of work. This helps prevent multitasking and ensures focused work.

5. **Eliminate Distractions:** Identify common distractions and take steps to minimize them. This may include turning off notifications, creating a dedicated workspace, or using website blockers.

6. **Set SMART Goals:** SMART goals are Specific, Measurable, Achievable, Relevant, and Time-bound. When setting goals, ensure they meet these criteria to increase your chances of success.

7. **Use the Two-Minute Rule:** If a task can be completed in two minutes or less, do it immediately. This prevents small tasks from piling up on your to-do list.

8. **Batch Similar Tasks:** Group similar tasks together and tackle them during the same time block. This minimizes mental context-switching and increases efficiency.

9. **Delegate When Possible:** Delegate tasks that others can handle, whether at work or home. Delegation frees up your time for more critical responsibilities.

10. **Set Boundaries:** Communicate your work hours and availability to colleagues, family, and friends. Establish clear boundaries to protect your personal time.

11. **Learn to Say No:** Be selective about accepting additional commitments. Saying no when necessary is crucial for managing your time effectively.

12. **Time Audit:** Periodically conduct a time audit to assess how you're spending your time. Identify areas where you can make improvements and eliminate time-wasting activities.

Time Management Tips:

- **Start Early:** Begin your day with a clear plan and tackle your most important tasks in the morning when your energy and focus are at their peak.
- **Use Deadlines:** Set self-imposed deadlines for tasks to create a sense of urgency and accountability.
- **Review and Reflect:** At the end of each day or week, review your progress, adjust your plans as needed, and celebrate your achievements.

- **Be Flexible:** While it's essential to have a schedule, be adaptable. Unexpected events can occur, so build some flexibility into your plans.
- **Practice Self-Care:** Allocate time for self-care activities, including exercise, meditation, and relaxation. These activities recharge your energy and reduce stress.
- **Continuous Improvement:** Continually refine your time management skills based on your experiences and evolving priorities.

Remember that effective time management is a skill that improves with practice. Experiment with various tools and strategies to discover what works best for you, and tailor your approach to align with your goals and values. Over time, mastering time management will help you reduce stress, increase productivity, and achieve a more balanced and fulfilling life.

Here are two case studies of individuals who transformed their lives through better time management:

Case Study 1: Sarah's Journey to Work-Life Balance

Background: Sarah was a successful marketing manager in a busy advertising agency. She was passionate about her work but found herself constantly stressed and overwhelmed. Her long work hours and frequent business trips left little time for her family and personal life.

Transformation: Sarah decided to take control of her time and achieve a better work-life balance. She implemented the following time management strategies:

1. **Set Clear Priorities:** Sarah identified her top work priorities and aligned them with her personal values. This helped her focus on projects that truly mattered and delegate or eliminate tasks that didn't contribute to her goals.
2. **Time Blocking:** She started time-blocking her workdays, allocating specific hours for meetings, creative tasks, and email management. This structure allowed her to work more efficiently and reduce distractions.

3. **Delegate and Empower:** Sarah began delegating tasks to her team members and empowering them to take ownership of projects. This freed up her time for strategic planning and reduced her workload.
4. **Set Boundaries:** She communicated her work hours to her colleagues and set boundaries on her availability during evenings and weekends. This protected her personal time and reduced work-related stress.
5. **Self-Care:** Sarah incorporated self-care activities like daily meditation, exercise, and spending quality time with her family into her routine. These practices helped her recharge and reduce stress.

Results: As a result of her time management efforts, Sarah experienced a remarkable transformation. She achieved a healthier work-life balance, reduced her stress levels, and strengthened her relationships with her family. Her improved efficiency at work also led to better outcomes for her team and increased job satisfaction.

Case Study 2: Mark's Journey from Procrastination to Productivity

Background: Mark was a college student who struggled with procrastination and time management. He often found himself cramming for exams and submitting assignments late, leading to stress and lower grades.

Transformation: Mark decided to take control of his time and improve his academic performance. He implemented the following time management strategies:

1. **Set Specific Goals:** Mark set clear academic goals, including grade targets and assignment deadlines. This provided him with a sense of purpose and motivation.
2. **Time Blocking:** He created a weekly schedule that allocated specific time blocks for studying, attending classes, and completing assignments. This structured approach prevented last-minute cramming.
3. **Break Tasks into Smaller Steps:** Mark learned to break down complex assignments into smaller, manageable tasks. This made it easier to tackle them gradually and avoid feeling overwhelmed.

4. **Eliminate Distractions:** He identified common distractions, such as social media and his phone, and used website blockers and apps to minimize them during study sessions.
5. **Use the Pomodoro Technique:** Mark implemented the Pomodoro Technique, working in focused 25-minute intervals followed by short breaks. This approach improved his concentration and productivity.

Results: Mark's commitment to better time management yielded significant improvements in his academic performance. He consistently submitted assignments on time, studied more efficiently, and achieved higher grades. He also experienced reduced stress and a greater sense of control over his academic responsibilities.

These case studies illustrate the transformative power of effective time management. By implementing strategic time management techniques tailored to their specific situations and goals, both Sarah and Mark were able to reduce stress, achieve better work-life balance, and improve their overall well-being and performance.

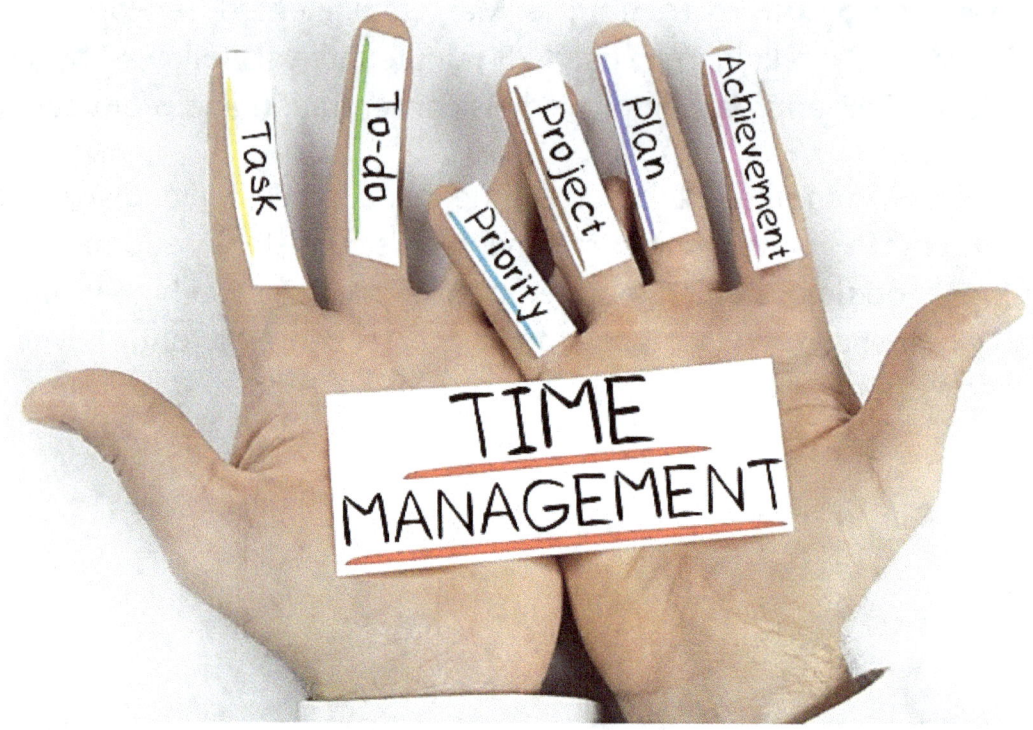

Fig 6: Time management is great asset in our daily lives

Chapter 6

Building Resilience

Harnessing Inner Strength: Building Resilience for a Stress-Free Life

Resilience is the ability to bounce back from adversity, adapt to challenges, and maintain emotional well-being in the face of stress. In this chapter, we delve into the importance of building resilience and provide practical strategies for developing this essential quality for a stress-free life.

Understanding Resilience:

Resilience is not a fixed trait but a skill that can be cultivated and strengthened. It involves the capacity to cope with adversity, manage stress, and maintain a positive outlook, even during challenging times. Resilient individuals are better equipped to handle life's ups and downs with grace and resilience.

The Role of Resilience in Stress Reduction:

Resilience is a key factor in reducing stress and promoting mental and emotional well-being. Here's why it's crucial:

1. **Emotional Regulation:** Resilience helps individuals regulate their emotions effectively, preventing them from becoming overwhelmed by stress and negative emotions.
2. **Adaptive Coping:** Resilient individuals are more likely to employ adaptive coping strategies when facing stress. They seek solutions, gather support, and maintain a problem-solving mindset.
3. **Positive Outlook:** Resilience fosters a positive outlook on life. It allows individuals to find meaning and growth in adversity, reducing the impact of stressors.
4. **Improved Stress Tolerance:** Resilience increases an individual's ability to tolerate stress. It builds emotional and psychological strength, making it easier to withstand challenges.
5. **Enhanced Problem-Solving Skills:** Resilient individuals are better at finding creative solutions to problems, reducing the sense of helplessness and stress.

Practical Strategies for Building Resilience:

1. **Develop a Growth Mindset:** Cultivate a belief in your ability to learn and grow from challenges. Embrace setbacks as opportunities for personal development.
2. **Build Social Connections:** Maintain strong social connections with friends and family. Social support is a powerful resilience-builder.
3. **Practice Mindfulness:** Regular mindfulness practice can enhance emotional regulation and increase resilience by promoting present-moment awareness and non-judgmental acceptance.
4. **Strengthen Problem-Solving Skills:** Develop effective problem-solving skills to address challenges more efficiently. Break problems into smaller steps and seek advice when needed.
5. **Self-Care:** Prioritize self-care activities such as exercise, healthy eating, and adequate sleep. A healthy body supports a resilient mind.
6. **Set Realistic Goals:** Set achievable goals and break them down into manageable steps. This prevents the feeling of being overwhelmed by large tasks.
7. **Cultivate Optimism:** Foster a positive outlook by focusing on positive aspects of situations, practicing gratitude, and challenging negative thought patterns.
8. **Embrace Flexibility:** Adapt to change and uncertainty by being flexible in your thinking and open to new perspectives and solutions.
9. **Develop Emotional Awareness:** Pay attention to your emotions and develop emotional intelligence. Understand and express your feelings effectively.
10. **Learn from Adversity:** Reflect on past challenges and consider what you've learned from them. This can help you approach future difficulties with greater resilience.
11. **Seek Professional Support:** If needed, don't hesitate to seek support from a therapist or counsellor. They can provide guidance and strategies for building resilience.

The Concept of Resilience and Its Importance in Dealing with Stress

Resilience is a multifaceted concept that refers to an individual's capacity to withstand, adapt to, and recover from adversity, trauma, or significant life challenges. It's the ability to bounce back emotionally and mentally after facing setbacks, stressors, or difficult experiences. Resilience is not an inherent trait but rather a skill and mindset that can be developed and strengthened over time. Here's a closer look at the concept of resilience and its paramount importance in dealing with stress:

Key Aspects of Resilience:

1. **Adaptability:** Resilient individuals can adapt to changing circumstances and remain flexible in their thinking and problem-solving approaches.
2. **Emotional Regulation:** Resilience involves the ability to manage and regulate emotions effectively, preventing them from becoming overwhelming or debilitating.
3. **Positive Outlook:** Resilient people maintain a hopeful and optimistic perspective even in the face of adversity. They focus on opportunities for growth and learning.
4. **Social Support:** Building and maintaining strong social connections is a critical component of resilience. Having a support network can provide emotional sustenance during difficult times.
5. **Self-Care:** Resilience is closely linked to self-care practices, such as prioritizing physical health, managing stress, and engaging in activities that promote well-being.

The Importance of Resilience in Dealing with Stress:

Resilience is of paramount importance in dealing with stress for several compelling reasons:

1. **Coping with Adversity:** Resilience equips individuals with the psychological tools to cope with and navigate adversity effectively. It helps them avoid becoming overwhelmed or succumbing to stress-related mental health challenges.
2. **Emotional Regulation:** Resilient individuals are better at managing their emotional responses to stressors. They can acknowledge their

feelings without being dominated by them, which prevents emotional burnout.

3. **Reducing Vulnerability to Stress:** Developing resilience reduces an individual's vulnerability to stress. Resilient people are less likely to experience chronic stress, anxiety, or depression in response to life's challenges.

4. **Enhancing Problem-Solving Skills:** Resilience fosters effective problem-solving skills, enabling individuals to approach stressors with a solution-oriented mindset rather than feeling helpless or defeated.

5. **Promoting Positive Coping Mechanisms:** Resilience encourages the use of positive coping mechanisms, such as seeking social support, practicing mindfulness, and engaging in self-care activities. These mechanisms are essential for stress reduction.

6. **Preventing Stress-Related Health Issues:** Chronic stress can lead to various health problems, including cardiovascular issues, weakened immune system function, and digestive disorders. Resilience acts as a protective factor, reducing the risk of these health complications.

7. **Fostering Post-Traumatic Growth:** In the aftermath of trauma or significant stressors, resilient individuals often experience post-traumatic growth, which involves personal development, increased wisdom, and a deeper appreciation for life's blessings.

8. **Enhancing Overall Well-Being:** Resilience contributes to overall well-being and life satisfaction. It promotes a sense of empowerment and control over one's life, reducing the negative impact of stressors.

Cultivating Resilience:

Cultivating resilience is an ongoing process that involves developing a growth mindset, building social connections, engaging in self-care practices, and seeking professional support when needed. By intentionally developing resilience, individuals can better manage stress, adapt to life's challenges, and ultimately lead healthier and more fulfilling lives. It's an essential skill that empowers individuals to not just survive adversity but thrive in its wake.

Developing resilience involves practicing specific exercises and techniques that enhance your ability to cope with stress and adversity. Here are some effective exercises and strategies to help you build resilience:

1. Practice Mindfulness Meditation:

- **Exercise:** Set aside time each day for mindfulness meditation. Sit comfortably, focus on your breath, and bring your attention to the present moment. When your mind wanders, gently return your focus to your breath.
- **Benefits:** Mindfulness meditation helps you become more aware of your thoughts and emotions without judgment. It enhances emotional regulation and reduces stress.

2. Keep a Resilience Journal:

- **Exercise:** Start a journal where you can record challenging situations you've faced and how you responded to them. Reflect on what you learned from each experience and how it contributed to your resilience.
- **Benefits:** Journaling promotes self-awareness, self-reflection, and a sense of mastery over adversity. It helps you identify patterns in your responses and areas for growth.

3. Develop a Growth Mindset:

- **Exercise:** Embrace challenges as opportunities for growth. When you encounter setbacks or failures, reframe them as learning experiences. Challenge negative self-talk and replace it with a growth-oriented perspective.
- **Benefits:** A growth mindset fosters resilience by encouraging a positive outlook and the belief that setbacks can lead to personal development.

4. Build a Support Network:

- **Exercise:** Cultivate and maintain strong social connections with friends and family. Seek emotional support and open up to trusted individuals about your challenges and feelings.

- **Benefits:** Social support is a powerful resilience-builder. It provides a sense of belonging, reduces feelings of isolation, and offers a source of comfort during tough times.

5. Engage in Physical Activity:

- **Exercise:** Incorporate regular physical activity into your routine, such as walking, jogging, or yoga. Exercise releases endorphins, which boost mood and reduce stress.
- **Benefits:** Physical activity not only contributes to physical well-being but also enhances emotional resilience by reducing the impact of stress hormones.

6. Develop Problem-Solving Skills:

- **Exercise:** Practice problem-solving by breaking down complex challenges into smaller, manageable steps. Set specific goals and create action plans to address them.
- **Benefits:** Effective problem-solving skills empower you to approach stressors with a sense of control and confidence, reducing feelings of helplessness.

7. Practice Self-Compassion:

- **Exercise:** Treat yourself with the same kindness and understanding that you offer to others. When facing adversity, practice self-compassion by acknowledging your suffering without self-criticism.
- **Benefits:** Self-compassion fosters resilience by promoting emotional well-being and reducing self-blame, shame, and perfectionism.

8. Seek Professional Support:

- **Exercise:** If you're facing overwhelming stress or struggling with resilience-building, consider seeking support from a therapist, counsellor, or mental health professional. They can provide guidance, coping strategies, and a safe space to explore your challenges.
- **Benefits:** Professional support can be invaluable in developing resilience, especially when dealing with trauma or complex emotional issues.

9. Foster Gratitude:

- **Exercise:** Regularly take time to express gratitude for the positive aspects of your life. Keep a gratitude journal or simply reflect on things you appreciate.
- **Benefits:** Gratitude enhances resilience by shifting your focus from adversity to positive aspects of life, reducing the impact of stressors.

Remember that developing resilience is a gradual process that requires ongoing effort and practice. By incorporating these exercises and techniques into your daily life, you can strengthen your resilience and better navigate the inevitable challenges and stressors that come your way. Building resilience is an investment in your mental and emotional well-being, ultimately leading to a more stress-free and fulfilling life.

Certainly! Here are two inspiring stories of individuals who have overcome adversity through resilience and determination:

1. Malala Yousafzai - Defying Extremism for Education:

Malala Yousafzai, born in Pakistan in 1997, faced tremendous adversity as a young girl. Growing up in the Swat Valley, she witnessed the rise of the Taliban and their strict restrictions on education, particularly for girls. Despite the danger, Malala was determined to pursue her education.

Adversity: At the age of 15, Malala was targeted by the Taliban for her advocacy of girls' education. In 2012, she was shot in the head while riding a bus home from school. The attack left her in critical condition.

Resilience: Malala not only survived the attack but also became a global symbol of courage and resilience. She continued her education in the United Kingdom and intensified her advocacy for girls' education worldwide.

Achievements: Malala co-authored the memoir "I Am Malala," which became an international bestseller. In 2014, she became the youngest recipient of the Nobel Peace Prize, and she has founded the Malala Fund, dedicated to promoting girls' education globally. Malala's resilience in the face of adversity has inspired millions and changed the conversation about the importance of education, especially for girls in underserved areas.

2. Nick Vujicic - Finding Purpose without Limbs:

Nick Vujicic was born in Australia in 1982 with a rare condition called tetra-amelia syndrome, which left him without limbs. Growing up, he faced immense physical and emotional challenges, including bullying and depression due to his disability.

Adversity: Nick's physical condition made daily tasks challenging, and he struggled with feelings of hopelessness and despair. He faced discrimination and cruelty from peers.

Resilience: Despite his challenges, Nick refused to let his disability define him. He developed a remarkable sense of resilience and a determination to live life to the fullest. He learned to perform everyday tasks with his feet and developed a positive outlook on life.

Achievements: Nick became a motivational speaker, sharing his story of resilience and perseverance with audiences worldwide. He founded the Life Without Limbs organization, which focuses on inspiring people to overcome adversity and find purpose. Nick's journey from despair to hope has touched countless lives, reminding us of the power of resilience and a positive mindset in the face of extreme adversity.

These stories illustrate the incredible strength of the human spirit and the capacity for resilience to overcome even the most challenging circumstances. Malala Yousafzai and Nick Vujicic serve as inspiring examples of individuals who have not only faced adversity head-on but have also used their experiences to make a positive impact on the world, emphasizing the importance of education, hope, and determination.

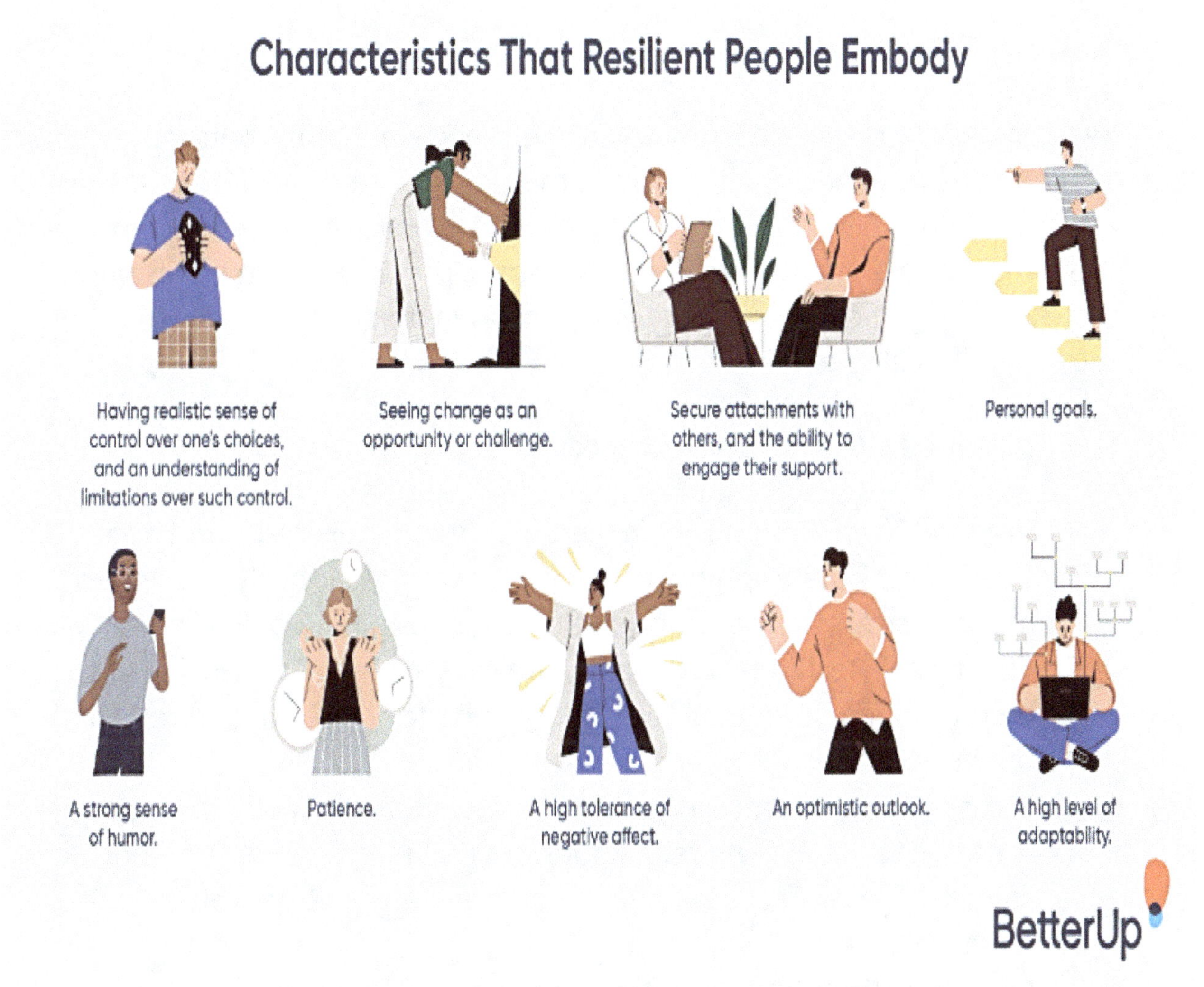

Characteristics That Resilient People Embody

Having realistic sense of control over one's choices, and an understanding of limitations over such control.

Seeing change as an opportunity or challenge.

Secure attachments with others, and the ability to engage their support.

Personal goals.

A strong sense of humor.

Patience.

A high tolerance of negative affect.

An optimistic outlook.

A high level of adaptability.

BetterUp

Fig. 6: Resilient and proper planning help relieve stress

Chapter 7

Understanding Healthy Lifestyle Choices

Elevate Your Well-Being: Nurturing a Stress-Free Life Through Healthy Living

A pivotal aspect of leading a stress-free life is making conscious and sustainable choices that prioritize your physical and mental well-being. In this chapter, we explore the significance of healthy lifestyle choices and provide practical guidance on how to cultivate a lifestyle that reduces stress and promotes overall health and vitality.

Understanding Healthy Lifestyle Choices:

Healthy lifestyle choices encompass a wide range of habits, behaviours, and decisions that influence your physical, mental, and emotional health. These choices include but are not limited to nutrition, physical activity, sleep, stress management, and social connections. Opting for healthy lifestyle choices can significantly enhance your resilience to stress and contribute to your overall quality of life.

The Role of Healthy Lifestyle Choices in Stress Reduction:

1. **Physical Well-Being:** A balanced diet, regular exercise, and adequate sleep contribute to physical health, boosting your body's ability to manage stress and reducing the risk of stress-related illnesses.
2. **Emotional Resilience:** A healthy lifestyle fosters emotional resilience by promoting emotional regulation, enhancing mood, and reducing the impact of negative emotions.
3. **Stress Management:** Engaging in stress-reducing activities, such as exercise and relaxation techniques, forms an integral part of a healthy lifestyle. These practices help you manage and mitigate stress effectively.
4. **Cognitive Function:** Nutrition and exercise play a crucial role in cognitive function, improving concentration, memory, and problem-solving abilities.
5. **Social Connections:** Building and nurturing social connections is a key aspect of a healthy lifestyle. Strong relationships provide emotional support and reduce feelings of isolation and stress.

Practical Strategies for Healthy Living:

1. **Balanced Nutrition:** Adopt a well-rounded and balanced diet rich in fruits, vegetables, whole grains, lean proteins, and healthy fats. Limit the consumption of processed foods, sugar, and caffeine.
2. **Regular Physical Activity:** Incorporate regular exercise into your routine. Aim for at least 150 minutes of moderate-intensity exercise per week, along with strength training exercises.
3. **Adequate Sleep:** Prioritize sleep by establishing a consistent sleep schedule and creating a restful sleep environment. Aim for 7-9 hours of quality sleep per night.
4. **Stress Reduction Techniques:** Practice stress reduction techniques like mindfulness meditation, deep breathing exercises, progressive muscle relaxation, or yoga to manage and alleviate stress.
5. **Time for Self-Care:** Dedicate time for self-care activities that rejuvenate your mind and body. This may include hobbies, creative pursuits, or simply moments of relaxation.
6. **Limit Screen Time:** Minimize excessive screen time, particularly before bedtime, as it can disrupt sleep patterns and contribute to stress.
7. **Hydration:** Stay adequately hydrated by drinking water throughout the day. Dehydration can impact mood and cognitive function.
8. **Social Connections:** Foster and maintain strong social connections by spending time with loved ones, engaging in social activities, and seeking support when needed.
9. **Regular Check-Ups:** Schedule regular check-ups with healthcare professionals to monitor your physical and mental health.
10. **Limit Alcohol and Avoid Substance Abuse:** Consume alcohol in moderation, and avoid substance abuse, as these can exacerbate stress and mental health issues.

Creating Sustainable Habits:

To make healthy lifestyle choices sustainable, start with small, manageable changes and gradually build upon them. Create a support system to help you stay accountable, and be patient with yourself as you adapt to a healthier way of living. Remember that the journey toward a stress-free life is a marathon, not a sprint, and every positive choice contributes to your well-being and resilience.

The Role of Nutrition, Exercise, and Sleep in Stress Management

Nutrition, exercise, and sleep are fundamental pillars of a healthy lifestyle that play a pivotal role in stress management. By understanding how each of these components contributes to your overall well-being, you can harness their power to reduce stress and build resilience effectively.

1. Nutrition:

a. Balanced Diet: Eating a well-rounded and balanced diet is essential for stress management. Nutrient-rich foods provide the body with the necessary vitamins, minerals, and antioxidants to support physical and mental health. A diet rich in fruits, vegetables, whole grains, lean proteins, and healthy fats helps regulate stress hormones and reduces inflammation.

b. Blood Sugar Regulation: Maintaining stable blood sugar levels is crucial for emotional well-being. Consuming complex carbohydrates, such as whole grains, and combining them with lean proteins and healthy fats helps prevent energy crashes and mood swings associated with fluctuating blood sugar levels.

c. Hydration: Dehydration can amplify stress and negatively affect mood and cognitive function. Drinking an adequate amount of water throughout the day is essential for optimal physical and mental performance.

d. Limiting Stimulants: Excessive caffeine and sugar intake can contribute to increased stress and anxiety. Limiting or moderating the consumption of stimulants can lead to a more stable and calm state of mind.

2. Exercise:

a. Stress-Reduction Hormones: Regular physical activity triggers the release of endorphins, the body's natural stress-relievers. Exercise stimulates the production of these "feel-good" hormones, which can boost mood and reduce stress.

b. Muscle Tension Reduction: Stress often manifests as muscle tension. Exercise helps alleviate tension by promoting relaxation and improving circulation, reducing physical discomfort associated with stress.

c. Improved Sleep: Engaging in physical activity during the day can lead to better sleep quality at night. Exercise helps regulate the sleep-wake cycle, making it easier to fall asleep and stay asleep.

d. Enhanced Resilience: Regular exercise builds physical and emotional resilience. It strengthens the body's ability to handle stress and recover more quickly from challenging situations.

3. Sleep:

a. Stress Hormone Regulation: Quality sleep is crucial for regulating stress hormones, particularly cortisol. Inadequate sleep can lead to an overproduction of cortisol, increasing stress levels.

b. Emotional Regulation: Adequate sleep supports emotional regulation and reduces irritability and mood swings. It helps maintain a positive outlook and reduces the emotional impact of stressors.

c. Cognitive Function: Sleep is essential for cognitive functions such as memory, concentration, and problem-solving. A well-rested mind is better equipped to manage stress and make sound decisions.

d. Restoration and Recovery: Sleep provides the body with an opportunity to recover and repair itself. This physical restoration contributes to overall well-being and resilience.

Incorporating these lifestyle factors—nutrition, exercise, and sleep—into your daily routine can significantly enhance your ability to manage and mitigate stress. To maximize their stress-reduction benefits, aim for consistency and gradual improvements. Small, sustainable changes in your diet, exercise routine, and sleep habits can lead to profound improvements in your physical and mental well-being, ultimately creating a solid foundation for a stress-free life.

Making healthier choices is a gradual process that involves conscious decision-making and the development of sustainable habits. Here's practical advice to help you make healthier choices in your daily life:

1. Set Clear Goals:

- Start by identifying specific health-related goals. These could include improving your diet, increasing physical activity, getting better sleep, or managing stress more effectively. Having clear objectives will give you a sense of purpose and motivation.

2. Make Small, Incremental Changes:

- Trying to overhaul your entire lifestyle all at once can be overwhelming. Instead, focus on making small, manageable changes one at a time. For example, start by adding a serving of vegetables to your dinner or taking a short walk after lunch.

3. Plan and Prepare:

- Planning and preparation are key to making healthier choices. Plan your meals and snacks ahead of time, and consider batch-cooking healthy meals for the week. Having nutritious options readily available reduces the temptation to make less healthy choices.

4. Practice Mindful Eating:

- Pay attention to what and how you eat. Avoid distractions like TV or smartphones while eating, and Savor each bite. This can help you become more aware of your food choices and prevent overeating.

5. Choose Whole Foods:

- Opt for whole, minimally processed foods whenever possible. These foods are typically higher in nutrients and lower in added sugars, salt, and unhealthy fats. Fill your plate with fruits, vegetables, whole grains, lean proteins, and healthy fats.

6. Stay Hydrated:

- Drinking enough water is essential for overall health. Carry a reusable water bottle with you and aim to drink throughout the day. Sometimes, the body can confuse thirst with hunger, so staying hydrated can also help with appetite control.

7. Practice Portion Control:

- Be mindful of portion sizes to avoid overeating. Use smaller plates and bowls, and pay attention to recommended serving sizes on food labels.

8. Find Physical Activities You Enjoy:

- Exercise doesn't have to be a chore. Find physical activities that you genuinely enjoy, whether it's dancing, hiking, swimming, or playing a sport. Consistency is key, so choose activities you look forward to.

9. Schedule Exercise:

- Just as you would schedule work meetings or appointments, block off time in your calendar for exercise. Treat it as a non-negotiable part of your day.

10. Get Adequate Sleep:

- Create a bedtime routine that promotes good sleep hygiene. Ensure your sleep environment is comfortable, quiet, and dark. Aim for 7-9 hours of quality sleep each night.

11. Manage Stress:

- Practice stress reduction techniques like mindfulness, deep breathing, or progressive muscle relaxation. Make time for hobbies and activities that bring you joy and relaxation.

12. Seek Support:

- Share your goals with friends or family members who can provide encouragement and accountability. Consider joining a fitness class or seeking the guidance of a registered dietitian or personal trainer if needed.

13. Monitor Your Progress:

- Keep a journal or use a tracking app to record your food intake, exercise sessions, and sleep patterns. Tracking your progress can help you stay on course and identify areas for improvement.

14. Be Patient and Forgiving:

- Understand that making healthier choices is a journey with ups and downs. If you have a setback, don't be too hard on yourself. Instead, focus on getting back on track and learning from your experiences.

15. Celebrate Your Successes:

- Acknowledge and celebrate your achievements, no matter how small they may seem. Each healthy choice is a step toward a happier, more fulfilling, and less stressful life.

Remember that adopting a healthier lifestyle is a lifelong commitment. It's about making choices that support your physical and mental well-being, reduce stress, and contribute to a higher quality of life. By taking small, consistent steps and staying mindful of your goals, you can gradually build a healthier and more balanced life.

Here are two testimonials from individuals who have successfully adopted healthier lifestyles, showcasing the positive impact it has had on their well-being and stress management:

Testimonial 1: Sarah's Journey to a Healthier Lifestyle

Sarah, a busy mother of two, struggled with stress and fatigue for years due to her hectic schedule and poor eating habits. She decided to make a change for the sake of her health and her family.

"I used to be constantly stressed out, juggling work, parenting, and household responsibilities. I often reached for fast food and sugary snacks for convenience, which only left me feeling more drained and anxious. I knew I had to do something different.

I started by meal planning and preparing healthy, balanced meals for my family. We incorporated more fruits, vegetables, and lean proteins into our diet. At first, it was a bit challenging to break old habits, but the positive changes in our energy levels and mood were evident within a few weeks.

I also began incorporating daily walks into our routine, sometimes with my kids. These walks became our quality family time, and we all started feeling more connected and less stressed. I made sure to prioritize sleep, creating a calming bedtime routine that helped me unwind.

Over time, I noticed a significant reduction in my stress levels. I felt more in control, had more energy, and was better equipped to handle the demands of daily life. Making healthier lifestyle choices not only transformed my own well-being but also positively impacted my family's health and happiness. It was the best decision I ever made."

Testimonial 2: Mark's Fitness Journey

Mark, a software engineer, struggled with a sedentary lifestyle, poor eating habits, and stress-related health issues. He decided to take charge of his health and incorporate regular exercise and better nutrition into his life.

"For years, my job kept me glued to a computer screen for long hours, and I had developed unhealthy eating habits and gained weight. I also felt overwhelmed by work-related stress, which was taking a toll on my physical and mental health.

I started by gradually introducing exercise into my daily routine. I began with short walks during breaks and eventually progressed to a regular workout regimen. This not only improved my physical fitness but also became an excellent stress relief outlet.

I also made conscious choices to improve my diet. I swapped out processed snacks for healthier options like nuts and fruits. I started cooking more balanced meals at home and limited my consumption of sugary drinks.

The transformation in my life was incredible. I lost weight, felt more energetic, and my stress levels reduced significantly. I discovered that regular exercise not only improved my physical health but also boosted my mood and mental clarity. It became a vital part of my stress management toolkit.

Today, I can confidently say that I've not only adopted a healthier lifestyle but also developed a deep appreciation for the positive impact it has had on my overall well-being. Making these changes has allowed me to better navigate life's challenges with resilience and a sense of empowerment."

These testimonials highlight how making healthier lifestyle choices can lead to profound improvements in physical, mental, and emotional well-being. By prioritizing nutrition, exercise, and stress management, individuals like Sarah and Mark have successfully reduced stress and enhanced their overall quality of life. Their stories serve as inspiring examples of the transformative power of healthy living.

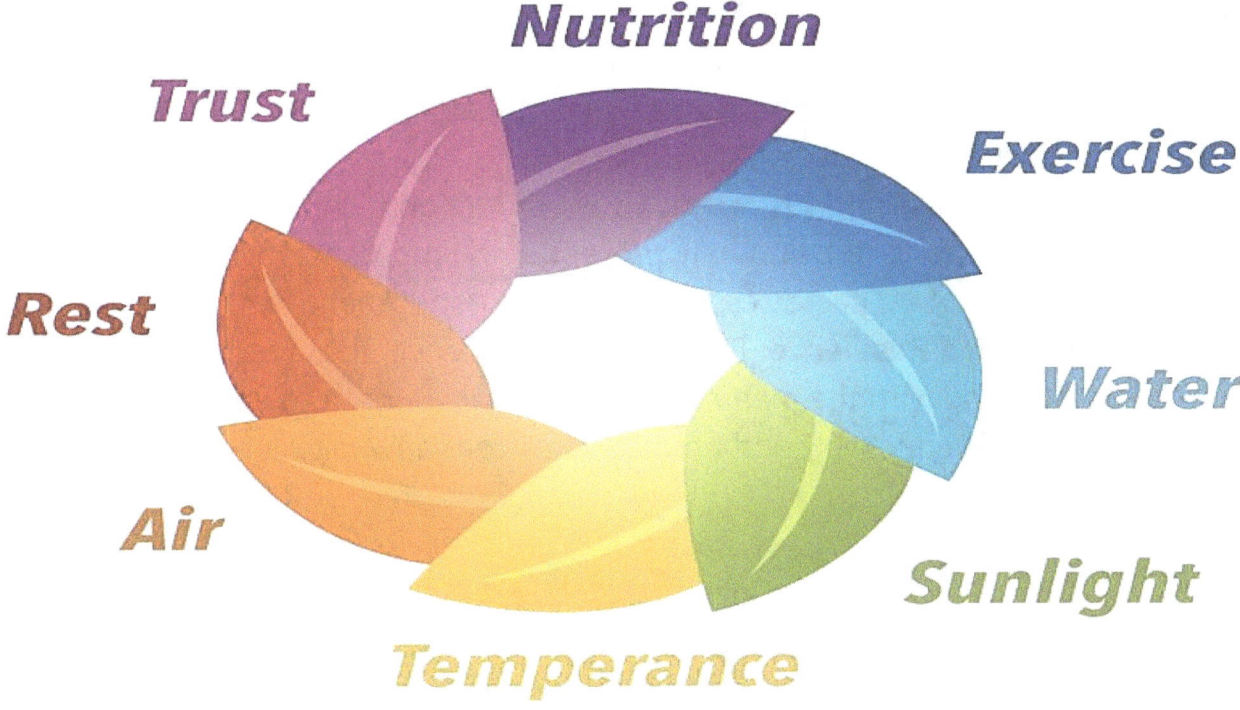

Fig.7: Living a better life style eases the chance of getting stress

Stress-reduction techniques

In this chapter, we will explore a variety of stress-reduction techniques that empower you to regain control of your emotions, thoughts, and physical responses when faced with stressors. These techniques, when incorporated into your daily life, can help you find tranquillity, build resilience, and ultimately live a more stress-free existence.

Understanding Stress-Reduction Techniques:

Stress-reduction techniques encompass a diverse range of practices and strategies aimed at managing and mitigating stress. They address the physical, emotional, and psychological aspects of stress, offering tools to bring balance and serenity to your life.

The Role of Stress-Reduction Techniques in Stress Management:

Effective stress-reduction techniques are instrumental in:

1. **Emotional Regulation:** They help you gain mastery over your emotional responses, preventing stress from overwhelming you and leading to heightened anxiety or mood disturbances.
2. **Physical Relaxation:** These techniques promote physical relaxation by reducing muscle tension, lowering heart rate, and regulating breathing patterns.
3. **Mindfulness and Presence:** Stress-reduction techniques encourage mindfulness and being fully present in the moment. This prevents rumination on past stressors or worries about the future.
4. **Enhanced Resilience:** By cultivating resilience, these techniques equip you with the mental and emotional strength to cope with stressors effectively and bounce back from adversity.

Practical Stress-Reduction Techniques:

1. **Mindfulness Meditation:**
   - **Technique:** Practice mindfulness meditation by focusing your attention on your breath, bodily sensations, or a specific object, all while gently acknowledging any wandering thoughts without judgment.
   - **Benefits:** Mindfulness meditation enhances emotional regulation, reduces anxiety, and promotes a calm and centered state of mind.
2. **Deep Breathing Exercises:**
   - **Technique:** Engage in deep breathing exercises, such as diaphragmatic breathing or the 4-7-8 technique, to slow your breathing and activate the body's relaxation response.
   - **Benefits:** Deep breathing reduces the stress response, lowers blood pressure, and promotes a sense of calm.
3. **Progressive Muscle Relaxation (PMR):**

- **Technique:** Systematically tense and then relax different muscle groups in your body. Start from your toes and work your way up to your head.
- **Benefits:** PMR reduces muscle tension, physical discomfort, and the physical symptoms of stress.

4. **Yoga and Tai Chi:**
   - **Technique:** Engage in yoga or tai chi, both of which combine physical postures with deep breathing and mindfulness. These practices improve flexibility, balance, and overall well-being.
   - **Benefits:** Yoga and tai chi promote relaxation, reduce muscle tension, and enhance mind-body awareness.

5. **Journaling:**
   - **Technique:** Keep a stress journal to express your thoughts and emotions. Use it as a tool for self-reflection, problem-solving, and identifying stress patterns.
   - **Benefits:** Journaling provides a healthy outlet for processing stress and gaining insights into its sources.

6. **Creative Expression:**
   - **Technique:** Engage in creative activities like art, music, or writing. These outlets offer a way to express emotions and thoughts that may be difficult to verbalize.
   - **Benefits:** Creative expression fosters self-expression, emotional release, and a sense of accomplishment.

7. **Spending Time in Nature:**
   - **Technique:** Spend time in natural settings, whether it's a park, forest, or by the sea. Connect with the soothing and grounding effects of nature.
   - **Benefits:** Nature immersion reduces stress, promotes relaxation, and enhances overall well-being.

8. **Guided Imagery and Visualization:**
   - **Technique:** Use guided imagery or visualization exercises to mentally transport yourself to a peaceful, calming place in your mind. Engage your senses to create a vivid mental picture.
   - **Benefits:** These techniques reduce stress by shifting your focus away from stressors and toward positive mental imagery.

Conclusion:

By incorporating these stress-reduction techniques into your daily life, you can cultivate emotional resilience, manage stress effectively, and embark on a path to a more tranquil and balanced existence. Each technique offers a unique approach to stress management, allowing you to discover what works best for you and ultimately leading to a more stress-free life.

Let's explore a variety of stress reduction techniques, including meditation, yoga, and deep breathing, each offering unique ways to manage and alleviate stress:

1. Meditation:

Technique: Meditation involves focusing your attention on a specific object, thought, or breath while eliminating distractions. It can be practiced in various forms, including mindfulness meditation, loving-kindness meditation, and transcendental meditation.

Benefits:

- **Emotional Regulation:** Meditation helps you become more aware of your emotions and develop emotional regulation skills. It can reduce anxiety, depression, and feelings of stress.
- **Stress Reduction:** Regular meditation practice reduces the production of stress hormones like cortisol, leading to a calmer mind and body.
- **Improved Concentration:** Meditation enhances your ability to concentrate and maintain focus, which can help you better manage stressful situations.

2. Yoga:

Technique: Yoga combines physical postures, controlled breathing, and meditation. There are various styles of yoga, including Hatha, Vinyasa, and Kundalini, each with its own emphasis on movement and meditation.

Benefits:

- **Physical Relaxation:** Yoga postures help release muscle tension and improve flexibility, reducing physical symptoms of stress.
- **Mind-Body Connection:** Yoga fosters a strong mind-body connection, helping you become more aware of physical sensations and emotions.
- **Stress Relief:** The mindfulness and deep breathing aspects of yoga calm the nervous system, making it an effective stress management tool.

3. Deep Breathing Exercises:

Technique: Deep breathing exercises involve taking slow, deep breaths to activate the body's relaxation response. The 4-7-8 technique, diaphragmatic breathing, and box breathing are common methods.

Benefits:

- **Reduced Physiological Stress:** Deep breathing slows the heart rate, lowers blood pressure, and relaxes muscle tension.
- **Stress Reduction:** These exercises are portable and can be practiced anywhere, making them a convenient tool for immediate stress relief.
- **Enhanced Oxygenation:** Deep breathing increases oxygen levels in the bloodstream, promoting a sense of clarity and calm.

4. Progressive Muscle Relaxation (PMR):

Technique: PMR involves systematically tensing and then relaxing different muscle groups in the body. This process helps release physical tension.

Benefits:

- **Muscle Relaxation:** PMR reduces muscle tension, which is often a physical manifestation of stress.

- **Stress Reduction:** By focusing on the physical sensations of relaxation, PMR can redirect your attention away from stressors.
- **Better Sleep:** Many people use PMR as a relaxation technique before bedtime to improve sleep quality.

5. Tai Chi:

Technique: Tai Chi is a mind-body practice that combines slow, flowing movements with deep breathing and meditation. It is often referred to as "meditation in motion."

Benefits:

- **Stress Reduction:** Tai Chi promotes relaxation, reduces muscle tension, and calms the mind.
- **Balance and Coordination:** The practice improves balance and coordination, which can boost confidence and reduce stress associated with physical limitations.
- **Mindfulness:** Like yoga, Tai Chi enhances the mind-body connection and cultivates mindfulness.

6. Guided Imagery and Visualization:

Technique: Guided imagery involves mentally visualizing a peaceful, calming scene or scenario. It can be done with the help of a guided meditation or simply through your own imagination.

Benefits:

- **Stress Distraction:** Visualization takes your mind off stressors and transports you to a serene mental space.
- **Emotional Calming:** Creating vivid mental images of tranquillity can evoke positive emotions and reduce stress.

- **Improved Focus:** Visualization exercises can enhance your ability to concentrate and remain present.

7. Mindfulness-Based Stress Reduction (MBSR):

Technique: MBSR is a structured program that combines mindfulness meditation with yoga and mindful awareness practices. It's often taught in group settings or through online courses.

Benefits:

- **Stress Reduction:** MBSR has been shown to reduce stress, anxiety, and symptoms of depression.
- **Increased Resilience:** By fostering mindfulness and awareness, this program helps individuals build emotional resilience to handle stressors more effectively.
- **Improved Well-Being:** MBSR can enhance overall well-being by promoting a greater sense of inner peace and acceptance.

Each of these stress reduction techniques offers a unique approach to managing and alleviating stress. The key is to explore and experiment with various methods to discover what resonates best with you and fits into your daily life. By incorporating one or more of these techniques into your routine, you can empower yourself to better navigate stress and lead a more balanced and stress-free life.

Here are step-by-step instructions for each of the stress reduction techniques mentioned:

1. Meditation:

- **Find a Quiet Space:** Choose a quiet place where you won't be disturbed.
- **Sit Comfortably:** Sit in a comfortable position with your back straight and your hands resting on your lap.
- **Focus on Your Breath:** Close your eyes and take a few deep breaths. Then, shift your attention to your breath. Notice the sensation of the

breath as it enters and leaves your nostrils or the rise and fall of your chest or abdomen.

- **Acknowledge Thoughts:** When your mind inevitably wanders, gently acknowledge any thoughts or distractions that arise without judgment. Bring your focus back to your breath.
- **Start with Short Sessions:** Begin with 5-10 minutes of meditation and gradually extend the duration as you become more comfortable with the practice.
- **Practice Regularly:** Aim to meditate daily, even if it's just for a few minutes. Consistency is key to experiencing the full benefits of meditation.

2. Yoga:

- **Choose a Style:** Select a yoga style that suits your preferences and needs. Beginners often start with Hatha or Vinyasa yoga.
- **Use a Yoga Mat:** Lay out a yoga mat or a non-slip surface for your practice.
- **Follow an instructor:** If you're new to yoga, consider following along with a beginner-friendly online yoga class or a local instructor.
- **Focus on Breath:** Pay attention to your breath throughout the practice. Coordinate your movements with your breath, inhaling and exhaling as you move between poses.
- **Start Slowly:** Begin with basic poses and gradually progress to more advanced ones as you become more comfortable and flexible.
- **End with Relaxation:** Always end your yoga session with a few minutes of Savasana (corpse pose), lying flat on your back and relaxing your body and mind.
- **Stay Consistent:** Aim to practice yoga regularly, whether it's daily or a few times a week, to experience its full benefits.

3. Deep Breathing Exercises:

- **Find a Quiet Space:** Choose a quiet place where you can sit or lie down comfortably.
- **Sit or Lie Down:** Sit in a chair with your feet flat on the ground or lie down on your back with your hands resting on your abdomen.

- **Breathe Naturally:** Begin by taking a few natural breaths to centre yourself.
- **Deep Breath In:** Inhale slowly through your nose, counting to four as you breathe in. Feel your abdomen rise as you fill your lungs.
- **Hold Your Breath:** Hold your breath for a count of four.
- **Exhale Slowly:** Exhale through your mouth for a count of four, allowing your abdomen to fall as you release the breath.
- **Repeat:** Continue this 4-4-4 cycle for several minutes, gradually extending the duration if desired.
- **Stay Relaxed:** Focus on your breath, and if your mind wanders, gently bring your attention back to your breathing.

4. Progressive Muscle Relaxation (PMR):

- **Find a Quiet Place:** Sit or lie down in a quiet, comfortable space.
- **Start with Toes:** Begin with your toes. Tense the muscles in your toes and hold for a few seconds, then release. Feel the difference between tension and relaxation.
- **Progress Upwards:** Move systematically through your body, tensing and then relaxing different muscle groups. Work your way up from your toes to your head.
- **Breathe Deeply:** As you release tension from each muscle group, take a deep breath and exhale slowly.
- **Focus on Sensations:** Pay close attention to the sensations of relaxation as you release tension from each muscle group.
- **Complete Relaxation:** Once you've gone through all muscle groups, focus on your entire body, feeling the deep sense of relaxation.
- **Practice Regularly:** Incorporate PMR into your routine as needed for stress relief or as part of your bedtime routine for better sleep.

Remember that these techniques may take time to become fully proficient. Be patient with yourself and practice regularly to reap the benefits. As you become more skilled, you can adapt and personalize these techniques to suit your preferences and needs.

Personal anecdotes can offer powerful insights into how these stress reduction techniques can transform lives. Here are two anecdotes illustrating the impact of meditation and yoga:

Meditation: Sarah's Journey to Inner Peace

Sarah had always been a high achiever, but the stress of her demanding job and personal responsibilities began to take a toll on her well-being. She struggled with anxiety and found it increasingly difficult to manage her emotions. Feeling desperate for a change, she decided to try meditation.

At first, sitting in silence and focusing on her breath was a challenge for Sarah. Her mind was always racing with thoughts of work, family, and the never-ending to-do lists. But she persisted, starting with just a few minutes each day.

Over time, Sarah noticed a remarkable transformation. Meditation became her refuge—a sacred space where she could quiet her mind and regain control over her emotions. She began to experience moments of deep inner peace and clarity that she had never known before.

As Sarah continued her meditation practice, her anxiety diminished, and her overall outlook on life improved. She felt more resilient in the face of challenges and was better equipped to handle stress. Meditation had not only transformed her emotional well-being but had also brought a profound sense of peace into her daily life.

Yoga: Mark's Journey to Physical and Mental Balance

Mark had spent years working in a high-stress job, sitting at a desk for long hours, and neglecting his physical health. His stress levels were through the roof, and he had gained weight, which only added to his stress and discomfort.

One day, Mark decided to give yoga a try, despite initial scepticism about its effectiveness. He started with beginner-level classes and was surprised to find himself enjoying the practice. The combination of gentle movements, deep breathing, and mindfulness had a profound impact on his physical and mental well-being.

With consistent yoga practice, Mark's body gradually became more flexible, and he shed some excess weight. But it wasn't just the physical changes that amazed him; it was the newfound sense of balance and calm that permeated his life.

Yoga became Mark's anchor in a sea of stress. It was during his yoga sessions that he learned to let go of the worries and pressures of his job. The deep stretches and mindful breathing allowed him to release physical tension and mental stress.

Over time, Mark's stress levels decreased significantly. He found himself more patient, focused, and resilient in the face of work challenges. Yoga had not only transformed his physical health but had also brought mental clarity and emotional balance into his life.

These personal anecdotes demonstrate the profound impact that meditation and yoga can have on individuals dealing with stress. Through consistent practice, these techniques can lead to inner peace, emotional resilience, and a renewed sense of balance, ultimately transforming lives for the better.

Personal anecdotes can offer powerful insights into how stress reduction techniques can transform lives. Here are two anecdotes illustrating the impact of deep breathing exercises and mindfulness meditation:

Deep Breathing: Emily's Journey to Calmness

Emily, a young professional, was no stranger to stress. The demands of her job and the pressure to excel often left her feeling overwhelmed and anxious. One day, after a particularly challenging week, she stumbled upon deep breathing exercises while researching stress management techniques.

With a racing heart and a mind filled with worries, Emily decided to give deep breathing a try. She found a quiet corner in her office, closed her office door, and sat comfortably in her chair. She followed these steps:

1. She took a slow, deep breath in through her nose, counting to four as she inhaled.
2. She held her breath for a count of four.
3. She released the breath slowly through her mouth for a count of four, feeling the tension leave her body.

Emily repeated this process several times, and with each breath, she felt a sense of calm wash over her. The racing thoughts began to slow down, and the physical tension in her body started to ease.

Over the following weeks, Emily made deep breathing exercises a daily practice. Whenever stress began to creep in, she took a few minutes to focus on her breath. The impact was profound. She found herself better able to handle workplace pressures, and her overall sense of well-being improved.

Emily's journey with deep breathing not only transformed how she managed stress but also gave her a valuable tool to navigate life's challenges with a sense of calm and control.

Mindfulness Meditation: David's Path to Clarity

David was a middle-aged executive who had always been driven by ambition. His career success had come at a price—chronic stress, anxiety, and a feeling of emptiness. He decided to explore mindfulness meditation after reading about its benefits in a magazine.

Sceptical at first, David decided to start small. He allocated just five minutes a day to mindfulness meditation. Here's how he practiced:

1. David found a quiet space in his home, away from distractions.
2. He sat in a comfortable position with his back straight and closed his eyes.
3. He focused his attention on his breath, gently observing the rise and fall of his chest.

David quickly realized how challenging it was to quiet his restless mind, but he persisted. With each session, he found it a little easier to let go of racing thoughts and simply be present in the moment.

Over time, David gradually extended his meditation sessions to 15 minutes and then 30 minutes a day. As he became more skilled in mindfulness, he noticed profound changes in his life. He felt more centred, less reactive to stressors, and more in tune with his own emotions.

Mindfulness meditation also opened up a deeper sense of purpose for David. He began to prioritize activities that brought him joy and fulfillment outside of work, further reducing his stress levels.

David's journey with mindfulness meditation not only transformed how he managed stress but also offered him a profound sense of clarity, purpose, and emotional well-being that had been missing from his life for years.

These personal anecdotes demonstrate how deep breathing exercises and mindfulness meditation can have a transformative impact on individuals dealing with stress. By incorporating these techniques into their daily lives, Emily and David found new ways to manage stress and improve their overall well-being, ultimately leading to a more fulfilling and balanced life.

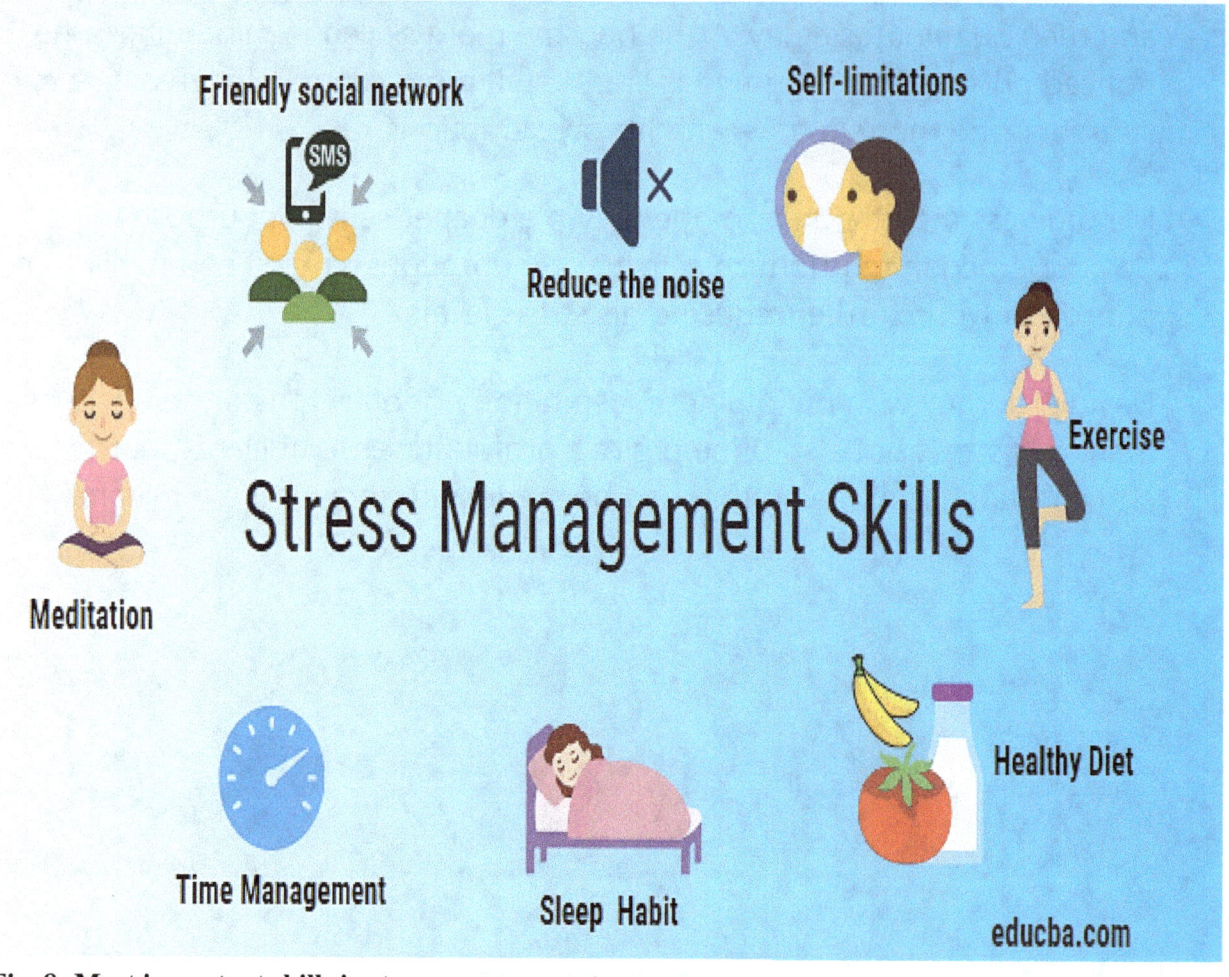

Fig. 8: Most important skills in stress management

Chapter 9

Understanding Positive Thinking and Mindset

The Power of Positivity: Cultivating a Stress-Resilient Mindset

In this chapter, we delve into the transformative influence of positive thinking and mindset on stress reduction. You will discover how adopting a positive outlook can enhance your resilience, fortify your mental well-being, and lead you on the path to a more stress-free life.

Understanding Positive Thinking and Mindset:

Positive thinking is more than just a feel-good notion; it's a fundamental shift in perspective and attitude. It involves consciously focusing on the bright side of life, finding opportunities in challenges, and nurturing a growth-oriented mindset.

The Role of Positive Thinking and Mindset in Stress Management:

1. **Emotional Resilience:** Positive thinking bolsters emotional resilience, enabling you to bounce back from setbacks and cope with stress more effectively.
2. **Optimism and Stress Reduction:** An optimistic outlook reduces the physiological effects of stress, such as elevated cortisol levels and increased heart rate.
3. **Problem-Solving:** A positive mindset enhances your ability to problem-solve, finding constructive solutions to stressors rather than dwelling on the negative aspects.

Practical Strategies for Cultivating Positive Thinking and Mindset:

1. **Practice Gratitude:** Regularly take time to reflect on and express gratitude for the positive aspects of your life. Keep a gratitude journal to record your blessings.
2. **Challenge Negative Thoughts:** Develop awareness of negative thought patterns and actively challenge them. Replace negative thoughts with more constructive and positive ones.

3. **Foster a Growth Mindset:** Embrace a growth mindset that views challenges as opportunities for learning and growth. Emphasize the belief that abilities and intelligence can be developed through effort and perseverance.
4. **Surround Yourself with Positivity:** Choose to spend time with people who radiate positivity and support your well-being. Limit exposure to negativity, both in relationships and media consumption.
5. **Practice Self-Compassion:** Treat yourself with kindness and understanding, especially during challenging times. Self-compassion helps counter self-criticism and fosters a more nurturing inner dialogue.
6. **Visualization:** Use the power of visualization to imagine successful outcomes and positive experiences. Visualizing a stress-free future can help make it a reality.
7. **Affirmations:** Create and repeat positive affirmations that resonate with you. These affirmations can serve as reminders of your strengths and resilience.
8. **Mindfulness and Positivity:** Combine mindfulness practices with positive thinking. Being fully present in the moment allows you to savour life's joys and cultivate a more positive outlook.

Conclusion:

Incorporating positive thinking and a growth-oriented mindset into your life can significantly impact how you perceive and respond to stress. By nurturing these qualities, you will not only build resilience but also create a more optimistic and stress-resistant approach to life's challenges. Embrace the power of positivity, and let it guide you on your journey to a stress-free life.

The Power of Positive Thinking in Reducing Stress

Positive thinking is a mindset and approach to life that emphasizes focusing on the constructive, hopeful, and optimistic aspects of any situation. While it may not eliminate stressors entirely, it has a powerful impact on reducing the harmful effects of stress and enhancing overall well-being. Here's how positive thinking can help in stress reduction:

1. Stress Perception:

- **Altered Perception:** Positive thinking can alter your perception of stressors. Instead of viewing them solely as threats, you can see them as challenges or opportunities for personal growth. This shift in perception reduces the emotional intensity of stress.

2. Stress Response:

- **Reduced Physiological Impact:** When you think positively, your body's stress response is less severe. Positive thoughts can lower cortisol levels (a stress hormone), decrease heart rate, and reduce muscle tension. This physical relaxation can counteract the damaging effects of chronic stress on the body.

3. Emotion Regulation:

- **Enhanced Emotional Resilience:** Positive thinking enhances emotional resilience, making it easier to cope with stress. Optimistic individuals tend to experience less anxiety and depression, even when facing adversity.
- **Improved Coping Mechanisms:** Positive thinkers are more likely to use constructive coping strategies, such as problem-solving and seeking social support, when dealing with stress. This leads to better stress management.

4. Cognitive Shift:

- **Reduced Rumination:** Positive thinking reduces rumination, which is the tendency to dwell on negative thoughts and experiences. Rumination can exacerbate stress and lead to anxiety and depression. Positive thinkers are more likely to let go of negative thoughts and focus on solutions.

- **Enhanced Problem-Solving:** Positive thinkers approach challenges with a problem-solving mindset. They are more likely to seek solutions and take action, leading to a sense of control over stressors.

5. Resilience Building:

- **Resilience Enhancement:** Positive thinking contributes to the development of psychological resilience. When you encounter setbacks or failures, a positive mindset helps you bounce back more quickly and adapt to new circumstances.

6. Social Support:

- **Positive Attraction:** Positive thinkers often attract and maintain strong social networks. These supportive relationships provide emotional bolstering during times of stress.

7. Physical Health:

- **Healthier Lifestyle Choices:** Positive thinkers are more likely to make healthier lifestyle choices, including better nutrition, regular exercise, and adequate sleep. These habits promote overall well-being and reduce stress.

8. Optimism and Longevity:

- **Longer Lifespan:** Numerous studies have suggested that optimism is associated with a longer lifespan and a reduced risk of chronic diseases. This longevity may be partially attributed to the stress-buffering effects of a positive outlook.

In summary, the power of positive thinking lies in its ability to reshape your perception of stress, modulate your body's physical response to stressors, enhance emotional resilience, and promote healthier coping strategies. By fostering a positive mindset and integrating positive thinking into your daily life, you can effectively reduce the impact of stress and work towards a more balanced and stress-free existence.

Changing negative thought patterns is a crucial step in promoting positive thinking and reducing stress. Here are some effective tools and strategies to help you transform negative thoughts into more constructive and positive ones:

1. Self-Awareness:

- **Mindfulness Meditation:** Regular mindfulness meditation can help you become more aware of your thoughts without judgment. This awareness is the first step in identifying and changing negative thought patterns.
- **Journaling:** Keep a journal to record your thoughts and emotions. This practice allows you to recognize recurring negative thought patterns and triggers.

2. Cognitive Restructuring:

- **Identify Negative Thoughts:** When you notice a negative thought, identify it and write it down.
- **Challenge Negative Thoughts:** Examine the evidence for and against the negative thought. Is there a more balanced perspective? What evidence supports a positive or neutral interpretation of the situation?
- **Replace with Positive Thoughts:** Once you've challenged a negative thought, replace it with a more positive or realistic one. For example, replace "I'm a failure" with "I made a mistake, but I can learn from it and improve."

3. Positive Affirmations:

- **Create Positive Affirmations:** Develop a list of positive affirmations that counteract your negative thought patterns. For example, "I am capable," "I am resilient," or "I am worthy of love and happiness."
- **Repeat Daily:** Repeat your positive affirmations regularly, especially in moments of self-doubt or stress. Over time, these affirmations can help rewire your thought patterns.

4. Visualization:

- **Visualize Success:** When faced with a challenging situation, take a moment to visualize a successful outcome. Imagine yourself overcoming obstacles and achieving your goals. This visualization can boost your confidence and reduce negative thinking.

5. Gratitude Practice:

- **Gratitude Journal:** Keep a gratitude journal to remind yourself of the positive aspects of your life. Write down three things you're grateful for each day, even if they are small.
- **Shift Focus:** When negative thoughts arise, consciously shift your focus to the things you're grateful for. This can help counteract negativity and improve your overall mindset.

6. Limit Negative Inputs:

- **Media Consumption:** Be mindful of the media you consume. Limit exposure to negative news or content that triggers negative thoughts.
- **Negative Influences:** Evaluate relationships that consistently bring negativity into your life. Consider spending less time with individuals who perpetuate negative thought patterns.

7. Positive Self-Talk:

- **Be Kind to Yourself:** Practice self-compassion. Treat yourself with the same kindness and understanding you would offer to a friend facing similar challenges.
- **Challenge Self-Criticism:** When self-critical thoughts arise, challenge them. Ask yourself if you would say the same things to a friend. If not, replace self-criticism with self-encouragement.

8. Professional Help:

- **Therapy:** If negative thought patterns are deeply ingrained or significantly impacting your well-being, consider seeking therapy or counselling. Cognitive-behavioural therapy (CBT) is particularly effective in addressing and changing negative thought patterns.

Remember that changing negative thought patterns takes time and practice. Be patient with yourself and acknowledge that it's normal to have occasional negative thoughts. The goal is to reduce their frequency and intensity and replace them with more positive and constructive thinking patterns. With consistent effort and the right tools, you can cultivate a more positive mindset and reduce stress

Certainly, here are two inspiring stories of individuals who adopted a positive mindset and transformed their lives:

1. Mary's Journey to Resilience:

Mary had always been an ambitious and driven individual, but a series of setbacks left her feeling defeated and consumed by negative thoughts. She had lost her job, faced financial difficulties, and experienced a personal loss all within a short period. These challenges led to overwhelming stress and a deep sense of hopelessness.

One day, Mary stumbled upon a book on positive thinking and decided to give it a try. She began by acknowledging her negative thought patterns and challenging them with more positive and realistic ones. Instead of dwelling on past failures, she focused on her strengths, skills, and the opportunities that lay ahead.

Mary also started practicing gratitude daily. She created a gratitude journal and made it a habit to write down three things she was grateful for each day. This simple act shifted her focus from what she had lost to what she still had.

Over time, Mary's positive mindset began to work wonders. She felt more resilient in the face of challenges and was better equipped to handle stress. She even started a small business, leveraging her skills and newfound optimism. As her business thrived, she realized that her positive mindset had been a driving force behind her success.

Mary's story is a testament to the transformative power of positive thinking. By changing her mindset and embracing gratitude, she not only overcame adversity but also built a more fulfilling and resilient life.

2. John's Journey to Self-Compassion:

John was a high-achieving executive who constantly pushed himself to excel in his career. While his drive led to success, it also came with a heavy dose of self-criticism. He was his own harshest critic, never satisfied with his accomplishments and always expecting more from himself.

One day, John's relentless pursuit of perfection took a toll on his physical and mental health. He experienced burnout, anxiety

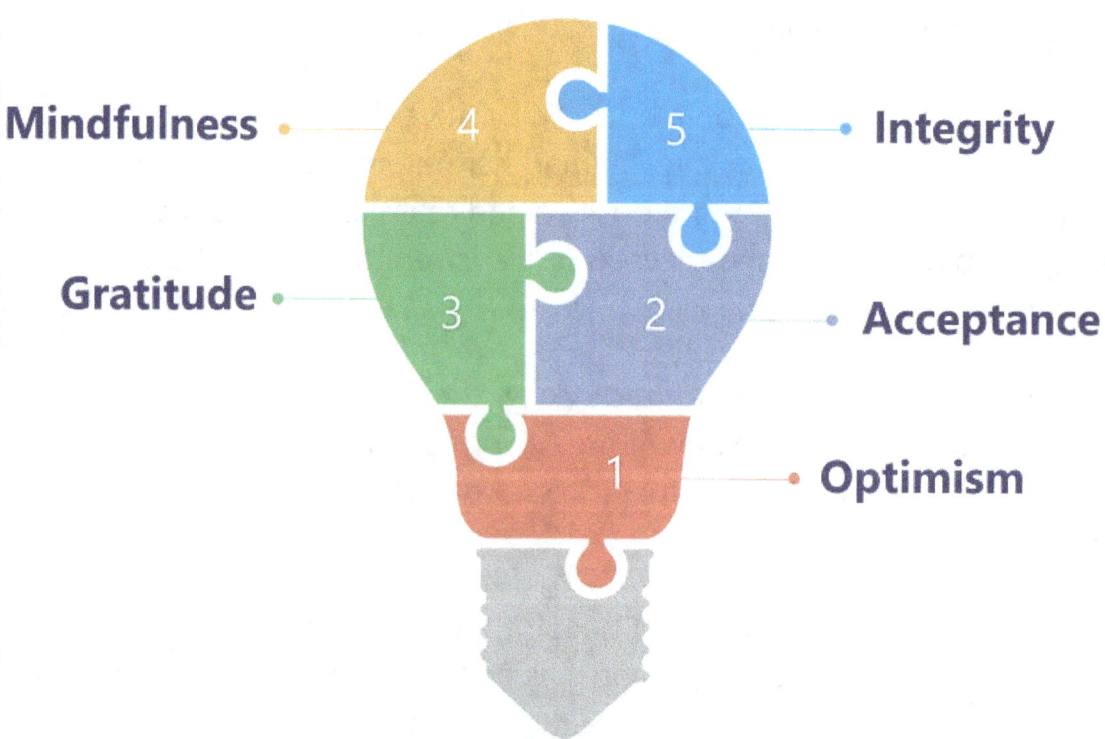

Chapter 10

The Vital Role of Relationships in Stress Reduction

In this chapter, we explore the crucial role that supportive relationships play in your journey to a stress-free life. You'll discover the profound impact of healthy connections on your mental and emotional well-being and learn strategies for cultivating and nurturing these relationships.

Understanding the Importance of Supportive Relationships:

1. **Emotional Resilience:** Supportive relationships provide emotional support during challenging times, bolstering your ability to cope with stress.
2. **Stress Reduction:** Sharing your feelings and concerns with trusted individuals can significantly reduce the emotional burden of stress.
3. **Enhanced Coping Strategies:** Supportive friends and family can offer valuable insights, advice, and different perspectives on how to deal with stressors effectively.
4. **Physical Health:** Strong social connections have been linked to better physical health, including a reduced risk of chronic diseases and improved immune function.

Strategies for Building and Nurturing Supportive Relationships:

1. **Open Communication:** Foster open and honest communication with your loved ones. Share your thoughts and feelings, and encourage them to do the same. Active listening is key to understanding each other better.
2. **Set Boundaries:** Establish clear boundaries in your relationships to protect your well-being. Boundaries help prevent stressors from negatively impacting your connections.
3. **Quality Time:** Dedicate quality time to spend with loved ones. Engage in activities that bring joy and create positive memories together.
4. **Conflict Resolution:** Learn effective conflict resolution techniques to address disagreements constructively and avoid escalating stress within your relationships.

5. **Empathy and Compassion:** Practice empathy and compassion in your interactions. Try to understand the perspectives and emotions of your loved ones, and offer support when needed.
6. **Social Support Network:** Cultivate a diverse social support network that includes friends, family, and other trusted individuals. Different people can provide various forms of support.
7. **Seek Professional Help:** If needed, consider seeking the guidance of a therapist or counsellor to improve your relationships and communication skills.

The Impact of Supportive Relationships on Stress Reduction:

In this chapter, you will encounter stories of individuals who have harnessed the power of supportive relationships to navigate life's challenges and reduce stress. These real-life examples will inspire you to strengthen your own connections and build a robust support system.

By investing in your relationships and surrounding yourself with supportive individuals, you can create a strong safety net that not only helps you manage stress but also enhances your overall quality of life. Building and nurturing these connections are essential steps on your path to a stress-free existence.

The Importance of Social Connections in Stress Reduction

Social connections, including relationships with friends, family, and a broader social network, play a pivotal role in stress reduction and overall well-being. Here's why social connections are crucial for managing and reducing stress:

1. Emotional Support:

- **Validation and Understanding:** Social connections provide a safe space for sharing your thoughts, feelings, and concerns. When you express your stress and worries to empathetic friends or family, you often feel validated and understood, which can alleviate emotional distress.

- **Catharsis:** Talking about your stressors with someone who cares can serve as a form of emotional release. Sharing your burdens can help you process and let go of negative emotions.

2. Stress Buffer:

- **Physiological Benefits:** Supportive social connections have been shown to reduce the physiological response to stress. Interactions with loved ones can lead to lower levels of stress hormones like cortisol and promote relaxation.
- **Stress Reduction:** Engaging in enjoyable and meaningful social activities can distract you from stressors and provide a sense of relief. Laughter and socializing trigger the release of endorphins, which are natural stress relievers.

3. Coping Strategies:

- **Problem-Solving:** Supportive relationships offer opportunities to discuss problems and find solutions. Friends and family can provide fresh perspectives and valuable advice on managing stressors.
- **Resilience Building:** Social connections enhance your capacity to bounce back from adversity. The emotional strength gained from supportive relationships contributes to greater resilience when facing life's challenges.

4. Cognitive Benefits:

- **Positive Influence:** Spending time with positive and supportive individuals can influence your thought patterns and encourage a more optimistic outlook. Positive social interactions can counteract negative thinking.
- **Mental Stimulation:** Engaging in conversations and activities with others stimulates your mind, promoting cognitive health and diverting your attention from stressors.

5. Motivation and Accountability:

- **Encouragement:** Supportive friends and family members can motivate you to maintain healthy habits and engage in stress-reducing activities such as exercise, relaxation, and self-care.
- **Accountability:** Having social connections who share your goals and aspirations can help you stay accountable to your stress-reduction strategies.

6. Sense of Belonging:

- **Emotional Fulfillment:** Feeling connected to others gives you a sense of belonging and emotional fulfillment, reducing feelings of isolation and loneliness—common contributors to stress.

7. Lifelong Benefits:

- **Longevity:** Studies have shown that individuals with strong social connections tend to live longer and enjoy better overall health. Social support is associated with a lower risk of chronic diseases and mortality.

8. Social Activities:

- **Engagement:** Participating in social activities or group hobbies not only fosters a sense of belonging but also provides an enjoyable way to de-stress and relax.

In summary, social connections are like a safety net that cushions the impact of stress in your life. The emotional support, stress-buffering effects, coping strategies, and cognitive benefits derived from strong relationships are essential components of a stress-free and emotionally resilient life. Cultivating and nurturing these connections is a valuable investment in your well-being and an effective means of managing and reducing stress.

Building and maintaining healthy relationships is essential for stress reduction and overall well-being. Here is advice on how to cultivate and sustain positive and supportive connections:

1. Communication:

- **Active Listening:** Practice active listening when others speak, showing genuine interest in their thoughts and feelings. Avoid interrupting and provide feedback to demonstrate your engagement.
- **Open and Honest Communication:** Foster an environment of openness and honesty in your relationships. Encourage discussions about feelings, needs, and concerns.
- **Conflict Resolution:** Develop effective conflict resolution skills. Approach disagreements with empathy and a willingness to find mutually agreeable solutions.

2. Boundaries:

- **Establish Boundaries:** Clearly define your personal boundaries and communicate them to others. Boundaries help protect your well-being and prevent stressors from negatively affecting your relationships.
- **Respect Boundaries:** Respect the boundaries of others as well. Acknowledge and honor their needs and limits.

3. Empathy and Compassion:

- **Empathetic Understanding:** Make an effort to understand the perspectives and emotions of your loved ones. Empathy fosters emotional connections and reduces misunderstandings.
- **Practice Compassion:** Be compassionate and kind in your interactions. Treat others with the same understanding and care you would want for yourself.

4. Quality Time:

- **Spend Quality Time Together:** Dedicate meaningful time to connect with friends and family. Engage in activities you both enjoy, fostering positive memories.
- **Unplug:** When spending time together, disconnect from digital devices and distractions to be fully present in the moment.

5. Support and Encouragement:

- **Offer Support:** Be there for your loved ones during difficult times. Offer emotional support, a listening ear, and practical assistance when needed.
- **Celebrate Achievements:** Celebrate each other's successes, no matter how small. Positive reinforcement strengthens relationships.

6. Self-Care:

- **Prioritize Self-Care:** Take care of your own physical and emotional well-being. When you are well-rested and emotionally balanced, you can contribute positively to your relationships.
- **Encourage Self-Care:** Encourage your loved ones to prioritize self-care as well. Support their efforts to maintain a healthy work-life balance and engage in stress-reducing activities.

7. Flexibility:

- **Be Flexible:** Relationships require flexibility and adaptability. Be willing to compromise and adjust to changing circumstances.
- **Respect Individuality:** Recognize and respect the individuality of your loved ones. Embrace their unique qualities and differences.

8. Apologize and Forgive:

- **Apologize When Necessary:** If you make a mistake or hurt someone unintentionally, apologize sincerely. Taking responsibility for your actions is a sign of maturity.
- **Forgive:** Practice forgiveness when others make mistakes. Holding onto grudges can erode relationships and increase stress.

9. Seek Help When Needed:

- **Professional Assistance:** If a relationship faces significant challenges or conflicts persist, consider seeking the guidance of a therapist or counsellor to improve communication and understanding.

10. Gratitude:

- **Express Gratitude:** Show appreciation for your loved ones regularly. Expressing gratitude strengthens bonds and fosters positive feelings.

11. Maintain Other Relationships:

- **Diverse Connections:** Maintain a diverse network of relationships. Different individuals provide varying forms of support, reducing the burden on a single relationship.

12. Be Patient:

- **Patience and Persistence:** Building and maintaining healthy relationships takes time and effort. Be patient with the process and persistent in your commitment to nurturing connections.

Remember that healthy relationships are a two-way street, and both parties need to invest time and effort. By following these guidelines, you can foster positive, supportive, and stress-reducing relationships that contribute significantly to your overall well-being.

Here are two stories of individuals who have improved their lives through stronger social networks:

1. Sarah's Journey to Recovery:

Sarah had always been a fiercely independent person. She took pride in handling her responsibilities on her own and rarely reached out for help, even during tough times. However, when a series of personal setbacks, including a health crisis, left her feeling overwhelmed, she realized that she needed support.

Sarah began by reconnecting with old friends and reaching out to family members she hadn't been in touch with for years. She hesitantly shared her struggles and vulnerabilities with them. To her surprise, they responded with empathy, love, and unwavering support.

As Sarah continued to nurture these rekindled relationships, she discovered the immense power of her social network. Her friends and family rallied around her, providing emotional support, practical assistance, and a strong sense of belonging. They helped her navigate her health challenges, offered a listening ear when she needed to vent, and encouraged her to prioritize self-care.

Over time, Sarah's health improved, and she found renewed strength in her connections. She realized that relying on her social network didn't make her weak but rather strengthened her resilience. Sarah's journey taught her that reaching out for support and fostering meaningful connections were essential for her well-being. Her life transformed as she embraced the richness of her social network, and she now enjoys a healthier and more fulfilling life.

2. John's Success Story:

John had always been ambitious in his career but often found himself overwhelmed by the demands of his job. His health began to suffer, and he felt isolated as he spent long hours at the office. Realizing the toll it was taking on him, John decided to prioritize his social connections.

He joined a local business networking group, not only to expand his professional network but also to build meaningful friendships. Through this group, he met individuals who shared his interests and values. They encouraged him to find a healthier work-life balance and offered support in achieving his career goals.

As John nurtured these connections, he started attending social events and participating in shared hobbies. These activities not only brought joy and fulfillment into his life but also reduced his stress levels. He found that his newfound friends provided a sense of camaraderie and understanding that he had been missing.

With the support and encouragement of his social network, John was able to make positive changes in his career and personal life. He achieved greater success in his profession while also maintaining a healthier work-life balance. The strong social connections he had built not only reduced his stress but also enriched his life in ways he had never imagined.

These stories highlight how building and strengthening social networks can lead to improved well-being, resilience, and a greater sense of fulfillment in life. Both Sarah and John learned that reaching out to others and fostering meaningful connections can be a transformative and empowering journey.

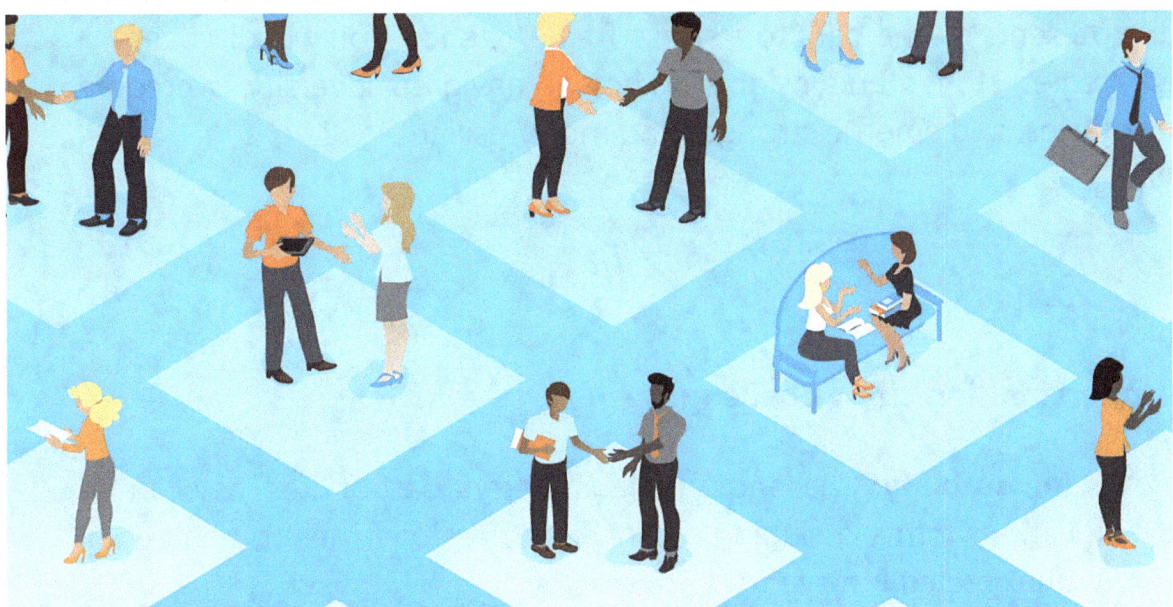

Fig. 10: Building healthy relationships in all life levels can greatly help in stress reduction

Chapter 11

Overcoming Obstacles

Facing Challenges and Thriving Amid Adversity

In this chapter, we delve into the inevitable challenges and obstacles that life presents on the path to a stress-free existence. You will discover strategies, stories, and insights on how to navigate adversity, overcome obstacles, and emerge stronger and more resilient.

Understanding Life's Challenges:

1. **Inevitability:** Challenges are an inherent part of life. They can take various forms, including personal, professional, health-related, or unexpected life events.
2. **Impact on Stress:** How you respond to challenges can significantly influence your stress levels. Avoiding or denying challenges can lead to chronic stress, while confronting them with resilience and adaptability can reduce their impact.

Strategies for Overcoming Obstacles:

1. **Mindset Shift:**
   - **Growth Mindset:** Embrace a growth mindset that views challenges as opportunities for learning and growth. Understand that setbacks are not failures but stepping stones to success.
   - **Positive Framing:** Cultivate the habit of framing challenges in a positive light. Instead of saying, "This is impossible," say, "This is a challenge I can overcome."
2. **Problem-Solving:**

- **Break It Down:** When facing a daunting challenge, break it down into smaller, manageable tasks. This approach makes problem-solving more achievable.
- **Seek Guidance:** Don't hesitate to seek guidance from mentors, experts, or supportive individuals who may have valuable insights into overcoming similar obstacles.

3. **Resilience Building:**
    - **Self-Care:** Prioritize self-care to maintain your physical and emotional well-being during challenging times. Exercise, adequate sleep, and stress-reduction techniques are essential.
    - **Adaptability:** Develop adaptability as a core skill. The ability to adjust to changing circumstances and find new solutions is invaluable.

4. **Social Support:**
    - **Lean on Your Network:** Reach out to your social support network during challenging times. Sharing your challenges and seeking emotional support can lighten the burden.
    - **Mutual Support:** Offer support to others when they face challenges. Mutual support strengthens relationships and provides a sense of purpose.

5. **Resilience Stories:**
    - **Real-Life Examples:** This chapter features inspiring stories of individuals who faced significant obstacles and emerged stronger and more resilient. These stories illustrate how resilience can be cultivated and applied in real-life situations.

Conclusion:

In this chapter, you will discover that obstacles are not roadblocks but opportunities for growth and personal development. By embracing challenges with a positive mindset, applying problem-solving skills, building resilience, and seeking support when needed, you can navigate life's hurdles and continue on your journey toward a stress-free life. Remember that your ability to overcome obstacles is a testament to your inner strength and resilience.

On the journey to a stress-free life, readers may encounter several common obstacles and challenges. Here are some of these obstacles and strategies to address them:

1. Negative Thought Patterns:

- **Obstacle:** Negative thought patterns can undermine efforts to reduce stress. Self-criticism, self-doubt, and rumination can intensify stress.
- **Strategy:** Practice cognitive restructuring to challenge and replace negative thoughts with more positive and constructive ones. Engage in mindfulness to become more aware of thought patterns and learn to let go of unhelpful thoughts.

2. Overwhelming Workload:

- **Obstacle:** A heavy workload or excessive responsibilities at work or home can lead to chronic stress.
- **Strategy:** Prioritize tasks and delegate when possible. Practice effective time management and set boundaries to maintain a healthy work-life balance. Seek support from supervisors, colleagues, or family members if necessary.

3. Relationship Conflicts:

- **Obstacle:** Conflicts in relationships, whether personal or professional, can contribute to stress.
- **Strategy:** Develop strong communication skills, practice active listening, and engage in conflict resolution when needed. Seek therapy or counselling for relationship issues if they persist.

4. Health Challenges:

- **Obstacle:** Health issues, chronic illnesses, or sudden medical emergencies can be significant sources of stress.
- **Strategy:** Focus on self-care and follow medical advice. Engage in stress-reduction techniques tailored to your health condition. Seek emotional support from healthcare professionals and loved ones.

5. Financial Stress:

- **Obstacle:** Financial difficulties, debt, or job loss can create substantial stress.
- **Strategy:** Create a realistic budget and financial plan. Seek assistance from financial advisors or counsellors if needed. Explore opportunities for additional income or financial assistance programs.

6. Lack of Support:

- **Obstacle:** Feeling isolated or lacking a strong support system can make it challenging to manage stress.
- **Strategy:** Cultivate social connections by joining clubs, support groups, or engaging in social activities. Seek therapy or counselling to address feelings of isolation or loneliness.

7. Procrastination:

- **Obstacle:** Procrastination can lead to the accumulation of tasks, resulting in stress due to impending deadlines.
- **Strategy:** Develop time management skills and break tasks into smaller, manageable steps. Set clear goals and deadlines to reduce procrastination tendencies.

8. Unrealistic Expectations:

- **Obstacle:** Setting overly high or perfectionist expectations for oneself can lead to stress when goals are not met.
- **Strategy:** Set realistic and achievable goals. Embrace the concept of "good enough" and practice self-compassion. Recognize that perfection is not a requirement for a stress-free life.

9. Loss and Grief:

- **Obstacle:** Experiencing the loss of a loved one can be emotionally overwhelming and lead to prolonged grief and stress.
- **Strategy:** Seek grief counselling or support groups to process your feelings. Allow yourself to grieve and express your emotions. Lean on your social support network during this challenging time.

10. **Lack of Self-Care**

Remember that overcoming these obstacles may require time, effort, and persistence. It's essential to seek professional help when needed, especially when dealing with complex challenges like mental health issues or significant life transitions. By addressing these obstacles with determination and a proactive mindset, readers can continue their journey toward a stress-free and more fulfilling life.

Here are strategies for overcoming common obstacles on the journey to a stress-free life:

1. Overcoming Negative Thought Patterns:

- **Strategy:** Practice mindfulness meditation to become more aware of your thoughts without judgment. Challenge negative thoughts by asking yourself if they are based on facts or assumptions. Replace negative thoughts with positive affirmations or more constructive thinking patterns.

2. Dealing with an Overwhelming Workload:

- **Strategy:** Prioritize tasks using methods like the Eisenhower Matrix (urgent vs. important) and delegate responsibilities when possible. Set clear boundaries to protect your work-life balance. Consider time management techniques like the Pomodoro Technique to boost productivity.

3. Resolving Relationship Conflicts:

- **Strategy:** Develop strong communication skills, including active listening and assertive expression. Practice empathy and try to understand the other person's perspective. Consider seeking couples or relationship therapy if conflicts persist and are affecting your well-being.

4. Managing Health Challenges:

- **Strategy:** Prioritize self-care practices such as regular exercise, a balanced diet, and adequate sleep to support your physical health. Work closely with healthcare professionals to manage health conditions. Engage in relaxation techniques like deep breathing or meditation to reduce stress related to health issues.

5. Addressing Financial Stress:

- **Strategy:** Create a budget and financial plan to manage your finances effectively. Explore debt consolidation or negotiation options. Seek assistance from financial advisors or credit counsellors. Consider additional income streams or side gigs to improve your financial situation.

6. Cultivating Support:

- **Strategy:** Actively seek social connections by joining clubs, support groups, or volunteering opportunities that align with your interests. Reconnect with old friends and make an effort to maintain relationships. Open up to trusted individuals about your need for support and connection.

7. Overcoming Procrastination:

- **Strategy:** Break tasks into smaller, manageable steps to reduce feelings of overwhelm. Set specific, achievable goals with deadlines. Use time management tools and techniques, such as to-do lists or time-blocking, to stay organized and on track.

8. Managing Unrealistic Expectations:

- **Strategy:** Set realistic and attainable goals, acknowledging that perfection is not necessary for success. Practice self-compassion and self-acceptance. Challenge the belief that you must meet excessively high standards to feel fulfilled.

9. Coping with Loss and Grief:

- **Strategy:** Allow yourself to grieve and express your emotions without judgment. Seek support from grief counselling or support groups where you can connect with others who understand your experience. Consider creating rituals or memorial activities to honour your loved one's memory.

10. Prioritizing Self-Care:

Remember that it's okay to seek professional help, whether through therapy, counselling, or coaching, to address specific obstacles or challenges that may be deeply rooted or complex. Overcoming obstacles on the path to a stress-free life is an ongoing journey that requires self-awareness, resilience, and a commitment to personal growth.

Here are some motivational quotes and anecdotes to inspire and encourage readers on their journey to overcome obstacles and lead a stress-free life:

Motivational Quotes:

1. "Obstacles don't have to stop you. If you run into a wall, don't turn around and give up. Figure out how to climb it, go through it, or work around it." — Michael Jordan
2. "The greater the obstacle, the more glory in overcoming it." — Molière
3. "Success is not final, failure is not fatal: It is the courage to continue that counts." — Winston Churchill
4. "Every adversity, every failure, every heartache carries with it the seed of an equal or greater benefit." — Napoleon Hill

5. "Strength does not come from winning. Your struggles develop your strengths. When you go through hardships and decide not to surrender, that is strength." — Arnold Schwarzenegger
6. "In the middle of every difficulty lies opportunity." — Albert Einstein
7. "Our greatest glory is not in never falling, but in rising every time we fall." — Confucius
8. "The only way to do great work is to love what you do. If you haven't found it yet, keep looking. Don't settle." — Steve Jobs

Motivational Anecdotes:

1. The Bamboo Story:

- Bamboo is known for its incredible strength and flexibility. In the first few years of its life, it appears to make little progress, as it primarily develops a complex root system underground. However, once it sprouts, it can grow up to 90 feet in just six weeks. This story reminds us that sometimes, progress is not immediately visible, and our efforts may take time to bear fruit. Patience and persistence are key to overcoming obstacles.

2. Thomas Edison and the Light Bulb:

- Thomas Edison made thousands of attempts before successfully inventing the electric light bulb. When asked about his "failures," he famously said, "I have not failed. I've just found 10,000 ways that won't work." This anecdote highlights the power of resilience and a growth mindset. Every setback is an opportunity to learn and move closer to success.

3. The Tale of the Two Wolves:

- A Native American grandfather tells his grandson that there are two wolves inside each of us, one representing anger, envy, and sorrow, and the other representing love, joy, and peace. The grandson asks which wolf wins, and the grandfather replies, "The one you feed." This story illustrates that our thoughts and actions determine our outcomes. Focusing on positivity and resilience can help us overcome obstacles and find inner peace.

4. The Butterfly's Struggle:

- A man once found a cocoon with a struggling butterfly inside. He decided to help the butterfly by carefully cutting the cocoon open. However, the butterfly emerged with a swollen body and weak wings. It was unable to fly. The man didn't realize that the struggle to break free from the cocoon was what the butterfly needed to strengthen its wings. This anecdote teaches us that sometimes, it's through adversity and struggles that we gain the strength needed to thrive.

5. The Rocky Road to Success:

- Many successful individuals, including J.K. Rowling, Oprah Winfrey, and Walt Disney, faced numerous rejections and setbacks before achieving their dreams. Their stories remind us that even when faced with seemingly insurmountable obstacles, determination and perseverance can lead to remarkable success.

These quotes and anecdotes serve as reminders that obstacles are an integral part of life's journey. How we approach and overcome them can define our path to a stress-free and fulfilling life.

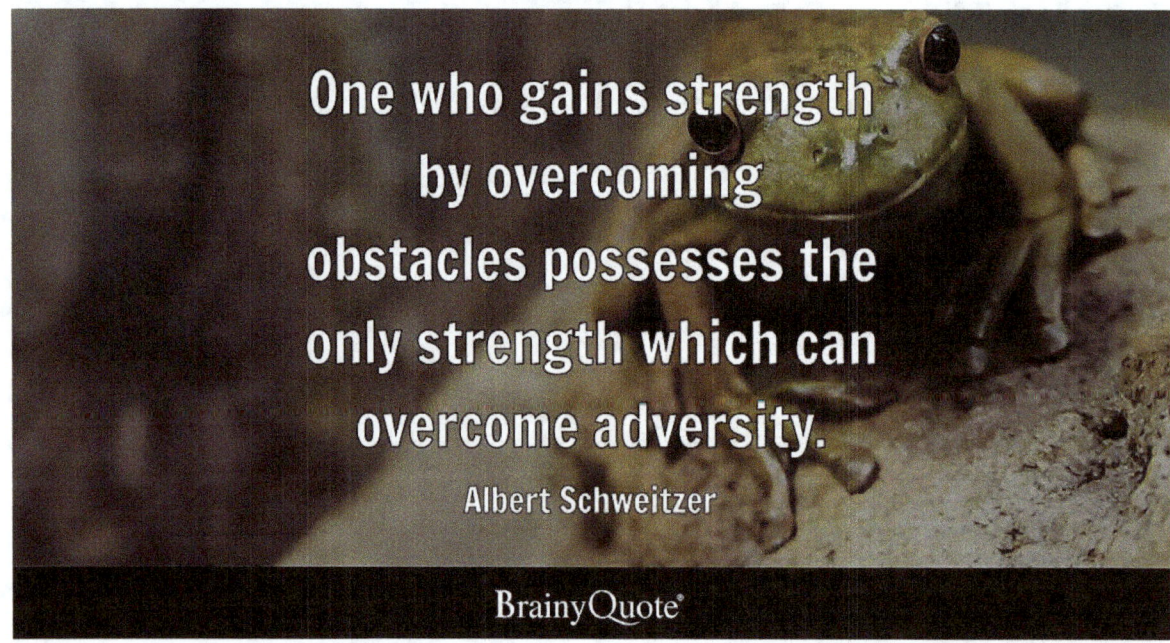

One who gains strength by overcoming obstacles possesses the only strength which can overcome adversity.

Albert Schweitzer

BrainyQuote

Chapter 12

Stress free life

Sustaining a Balanced and Stress-Free Existence

In this final chapter, we explore the art of maintaining a stress-free life once you've achieved it. A stress-free life is not a one-time destination but an ongoing journey. Here, we offer insights, strategies, and practical tips to help you sustain your newfound balance and well-being.

Embracing Stress-Free Living as a Lifestyle:

1. **Mindful Living:** Continue to practice mindfulness and self-awareness. Regularly check in with your emotions, thoughts, and stress levels. Mindfulness will help you stay attuned to your needs and address stress before it escalates.
2. **Boundaries:** Maintain and reinforce the boundaries you've established. Protect your time, energy, and well-being by setting clear limits in both your personal and professional life.

Staying Resilient:

3. **Resilience Building:** Keep building your resilience. Challenges and stressors will inevitably arise, but your resilience will empower you to navigate them with grace and adaptability.
4. **Stress Reduction Techniques:** Continue to practice stress-reduction techniques such as meditation, deep breathing, or yoga. Make them a regular part of your routine to prevent stress from accumulating.

Nurturing Relationships:

5. **Social Connections:** Prioritize your social connections and maintain a strong support network. Nurture your relationships through regular communication, quality time, and emotional support.
6. **Supportive Environment:** Surround yourself with people who uplift and inspire you. Create a positive and supportive environment that reinforces your commitment to a stress-free life.

Healthy Lifestyle Choices:

7. **Nutrition:** Continue making healthy food choices that nourish your body and mind. A balanced diet plays a significant role in stress management.
8. **Physical Activity:** Maintain a regular exercise routine. Physical activity not only reduces stress but also boosts your mood and overall well-being.
9. **Sleep Hygiene:** Prioritize quality sleep. Establish a sleep routine and create a comfortable sleep environment to ensure restorative rest.

Positive Mindset:

10. **Positive Thinking:** Continue cultivating a positive mindset. Challenge negative thought patterns and maintain a focus on gratitude and optimism.
11. **Self-Compassion:** Practice self-compassion and self-acceptance. Be kind to yourself and acknowledge that setbacks are a natural part of life.

Adaptability and Growth:

12. **Flexibility:** Embrace change and adaptability as a way of life. Life is dynamic, and your ability to adjust to new circumstances will contribute to your stress resilience.
13. **Lifelong Learning:** Stay curious and engaged in lifelong learning. Seek personal and professional growth opportunities to maintain a sense of purpose and fulfillment.

Prioritizing Self-Care:

14. **Regular Self-Care:** Self-care should not be sporadic but a consistent practice. Dedicate time each day or week for activities that rejuvenate and replenish your energy.

Reflecting on Your Journey:

15. **Periodic Reflection:** Periodically reflect on your stress-free journey. Celebrate your successes and acknowledge your growth. Revisit your goals and adjust them as needed.

Seeking Help When Needed:

16. **Professional Support:** Don't hesitate to seek professional support or therapy if you encounter significant challenges or experience a resurgence of stress. Seeking help is a sign of strength, not weakness.

Inspiring Others:

17. **Share Your Journey:** Share your experiences and insights with others. Inspire and support those around you in their quest for a stress-free life.

In this final chapter, you will find guidance on how to make stress-free living a sustainable and fulfilling lifestyle. Remember that maintaining a stress-free life requires ongoing effort and a commitment to your well-being. By incorporating these strategies into your daily life, you can continue to enjoy the benefits of reduced stress and increased happiness for years to come.

Here are the key takeaways from the book "How to Live a Stress-Free Life":

1. **Understanding Stress:**
   - Stress is a natural response to life's challenges, but it can become harmful when chronic and unmanaged.
2. **Positive vs. Negative Stress:**
   - Distinguish between positive stress (eustress) that motivates and negative stress (distress) that harms your health and well-being.
3. **Identifying Stressors:**

- Recognize the sources of your stress, both external and internal, to address them effectively.

4. **The Mind-Body Connection:**
   - Understand the profound impact of stress on your physical and mental health, and how to promote wellness through stress management.

5. **The Power of Mindfulness:**
   - Embrace mindfulness as a tool for reducing stress, improving focus, and enhancing overall well-being.

6. **Time Management and Prioritization:**
   - Effective time management and setting priorities are crucial for reducing stress and achieving a work-life balance.

7. **Building Resilience:**
   - Develop resilience to bounce back from adversity and challenges, strengthening your ability to cope with stress.

8. **Healthy Lifestyle Choices:**
   - Nutrition, exercise, and sleep play significant roles in managing stress and promoting well-being.

9. **Stress-Reduction Techniques:**
   - Explore various stress reduction techniques, including meditation, yoga, and deep breathing, to find what works best for you.

10. **Positive Thinking and Mindset:**
   - Adopt a positive mindset to reframe negative thoughts, manage stress, and increase overall optimism.

11. **Building Supportive Relationships:**
   - Foster and maintain positive relationships as they provide emotional support and enhance resilience.

12. **Overcoming Obstacles:**
   - Learn to navigate common obstacles on the path to a stress-free life with resilience and determination.

13. **Maintaining a Stress-Free Life:**
   - Sustaining a stress-free life involves continuous self-care, mindfulness, and maintaining a positive mindset.

14. **Inspiring Others:**
   - Share your experiences and insights to inspire and support others on their journey to a stress-free life.

Overall, the book emphasizes that living a stress-free life is a dynamic and achievable goal. It's not about eliminating all stress but managing it effectively and adopting a holistic approach to well-being. By implementing the strategies and practices outlined in the book, readers can enhance their quality of life, reduce stress, and embrace a more balanced and fulfilling existence.

Maintaining a stress-free life is an ongoing journey that requires commitment and mindfulness. Here's a roadmap to help you sustain a stress-free and balanced existence:

1. **Embrace Mindfulness and Self-Awareness:**

   - **Daily Practice:** Continue practicing mindfulness and self-awareness daily. Dedicate time for meditation, deep breathing, or other mindfulness exercises.
   - **Regular Check-Ins:** Periodically assess your stress levels, emotions, and well-being. Adjust your routines and self-care practices as needed.

2. **Maintain Boundaries:**

   - **Consistency:** Keep enforcing and respecting the boundaries you've established in your personal and professional life. Protect your time and energy.
   - **Reevaluate:** Periodically review your boundaries to ensure they align with your evolving needs and circumstances.

3. **Nurture Resilience:**

   - **Lifelong Growth:** Maintain a growth mindset and a commitment to resilience. Understand that challenges are opportunities for learning and growth.
   - **Practice Resilience:** Apply your resilience skills when facing adversity or setbacks. Remind yourself of past successes in overcoming obstacles.

4. **Cultivate Relationships:**

- **Prioritize Connections:** Continue nurturing your social connections. Dedicate time to spend with loved ones and maintain open communication.
- **Mutual Support:** Offer support to others when they face challenges. Strengthen your social network by being a source of positivity and encouragement.

5. **Healthy Lifestyle Choices:**

- **Consistent Habits:** Maintain a balanced diet, regular exercise, and sufficient sleep as essential components of stress management.
- **Regular Check-Ups:** Schedule periodic health check-ups to monitor your physical well-being and address any potential issues proactively.

6. **Positive Mindset:**

- **Daily Affirmations:** Incorporate positive affirmations and gratitude practices into your daily routine. Challenge and reframe negative thoughts promptly.
- **Self-Compassion:** Practice self-compassion and self-acceptance. Be kind to yourself, especially during challenging times.

7. **Adaptability and Growth:**

- **Embrace Change:** Welcome change and adaptability as a part of life. Cultivate a flexible mindset that enables you to adjust to new circumstances.
- **Lifelong Learning:** Continue seeking opportunities for personal and professional growth. Engage in learning activities that stimulate your mind and interests.

8. **Prioritize Self-Care:**

- **Scheduled Self-Care:** Integrate self-care practices into your daily, weekly, and monthly routines. Dedicate time for relaxation, hobbies, and activities that bring you joy.

9. Reflect and Revisit:

- **Periodic Reflection:** Reflect on your journey to stress-free living. Celebrate your achievements and recognize your growth.
- **Goal Adjustment:** Revisit your goals and aspirations periodically. Adjust them as needed to align with your evolving values and priorities.

10. Seek Professional Support

11. Inspire Others:

Remember that maintaining a stress-free life is an ongoing process, not a destination. The key is to stay mindful, prioritize self-care, and adapt to life's changes with resilience and a positive outlook. By following this roadmap, you can continue to enjoy the benefits of reduced stress and an overall more fulfilling and balanced existence.

To all the readers who have embarked on the journey towards a stress-free life, I want to extend my heartfelt encouragement and support. Your commitment to improving your well-being and pursuing a balanced, stress-free existence is a remarkable endeavour, and it's one that can bring about profound positive changes in your life.

As you progress on this path, remember these essential words of encouragement:

1. You've Already Taken the First Step:

- By picking up this book and dedicating your time to understanding and implementing strategies for a stress-free life, you've already taken a significant step forward. Acknowledge and celebrate this initial commitment.

2. Embrace Patience and Perseverance:

- Achieving and maintaining a stress-free life is not a quick fix; it's a lifelong journey. There will be days when you face setbacks and challenges. Understand that these moments are opportunities for growth and resilience-building. Be patient with yourself and persevere through the tough times.

3. Prioritize Self-Care:

- Self-care is not a luxury but a necessity on your journey. Consistently prioritize self-care practices that rejuvenate your mind, body, and spirit. Make them non-negotiable in your daily routine.

4. Cherish Your Support System:

- Lean on your social support network. Your friends, family, and loved ones are there to encourage and uplift you. Share your experiences and progress with them, and allow their support to strengthen your resolve.

5. Embrace Flexibility and Adaptability:

- Life is dynamic, and change is inevitable. Embrace adaptability as a way of life. Your ability to adjust to new circumstances and navigate challenges will be crucial in maintaining a stress-free existence.

6. Reflect on Your Journey:

- Periodically take time to reflect on how far you've come. Celebrate your successes, no matter how small they may seem. Recognize the positive changes in your life and use them as motivation to keep moving forward.

7. Share Your Wisdom:

- As you continue on your path to a stress-free life, consider sharing your experiences and insights with others. Your journey can inspire and support those around you who may be seeking the same balance and well-being.

8. Seek Professional Support When Needed:

- Remember that seeking professional support, whether through therapy, counselling, or coaching, is a sign of strength, not weakness. Don't hesitate to reach out when you encounter significant challenges or setbacks.

9. Your Journey is Worth It:

- Lastly, always remind yourself that your journey towards a stress-free life is worth every effort. The benefits extend far beyond the absence of stress. It's about finding a profound sense of peace, happiness, and fulfillment in your everyday existence.

So, keep moving forward with determination, resilience, and an unwavering belief in your ability to live a stress-free life. The road may have its twists and turns, but the destination—lasting well-being and contentment—is well worth the journey. You are capable, and you've already demonstrated your commitment to a brighter and more peaceful future. Continue on, and may your path be filled with joy and fulfillment.

Conclusion: A Stress-Free Life Awaits

In closing, I want to emphasize that a stress-free life is not an unattainable dream; it's a reality that can be yours with commitment, self-care, and the right mindset. The journey outlined in this book has equipped you with the knowledge, strategies, and inspiration needed to embark on this transformative path.

Remember that stress is a part of life, but it doesn't have to define your life. By understanding the nature of stress, identifying your stressors, and cultivating resilience, you have the power to reduce its impact and enjoy a more balanced and fulfilling existence.

Throughout the chapters, you've explored the significance of mindfulness, time management, positive thinking, healthy lifestyle choices, and the role of supportive relationships in stress management. You've learned how to overcome obstacles and maintain your newfound well-being as a lifestyle.

As you continue your journey towards a stress-free life, embrace patience, self-compassion, and adaptability. Know that setbacks are opportunities for growth, and every step forward brings you closer to your goal.

Your well-being matters, and you deserve a life filled with peace, joy, and contentment. Your commitment to this journey is a testament to your inner strength and your belief in the possibility of a stress-free life.

So, take these lessons and insights with you as you move forward. You have the tools, the resilience, and the support to create a life free from the burdens of chronic stress. It's a journey worth taking, and the destination is a brighter, more peaceful, and truly fulfilling life.

May you find the balance and tranquillity you seek, and may your days be filled with the serenity that comes from living a stress-free life. The path is yours to follow, and your journey continues with each step you take towards a brighter tomorrow.

The transformation that readers can achieve by following the advice in this book is nothing short of remarkable. By embracing the principles, strategies, and practices outlined within these pages, readers have the potential to undergo profound and positive changes in their lives.

Here's a reflection on the transformation readers can expect:

1. Stress Reduction and Improved Well-Being:

- Readers can expect a significant reduction in stress levels. By understanding the sources of stress and implementing stress-reduction techniques, they can experience a newfound sense of calm and serenity.

2. Enhanced Resilience:

- Through the exploration of resilience-building exercises and strategies, readers can become more resilient in the face of life's challenges. They will learn to bounce back from setbacks with grace and adaptability.

3. Better Time Management and Work-Life Balance:

- Implementing time management tools and techniques can lead to improved productivity and a healthier work-life balance. Readers can regain control over their time, allowing for more meaningful pursuits and relaxation.

4. Positive Mindset and Self-Compassion:

- Readers can cultivate a positive mindset and develop self-compassion. They will learn to challenge negative thought patterns, embrace optimism, and treat themselves with kindness, even in the face of difficulties.

5. Healthier Lifestyle Choices:

- By prioritizing nutrition, exercise, and sleep, readers can expect improvements in their physical health. These choices not only reduce stress but also boost overall well-being.

6. Stronger Social Connections:

- As readers invest in nurturing their relationships and building a supportive network, they can experience deeper connections and a stronger sense of belonging. These connections provide emotional support and enhance overall happiness.

7. Increased Self-Awareness:

- Through regular mindfulness practice, readers can become more self-aware. They will gain insight into their thoughts, emotions, and behaviours, leading to better self-management and emotional regulation.

8. Lifelong Learning and Personal Growth:

- Readers can look forward to a lifetime of learning and personal growth. By staying curious and open to new experiences, they will continue to evolve as individuals, finding fulfillment in lifelong exploration.

9. A Stress-Free Lifestyle as a Reality:

- Ultimately, readers can achieve the dream of a stress-free life. While stress is a natural part of life, they will have the knowledge and tools to manage it effectively, ensuring that it no longer dominates their existence.

The transformation readers can achieve is not only about the absence of stress but also about experiencing a profound sense of well-being, balance, and fulfillment in their everyday lives. By following the guidance and practices in this book, readers can create a future marked by tranquillity, resilience, and a deep appreciation for the beauty of a stress-free existence.

In closing, I want to offer you a final dose of encouragement and motivation on your journey towards a stress-free life. Remember that you possess the inner strength and resilience needed to transform your life, and every step you take is a step closer to a brighter, more peaceful future.

1. You are Capable:

- Believe in your capabilities and your capacity for growth. You have already demonstrated your commitment to change by seeking out this knowledge and guidance.

2. Embrace Progress Over Perfection:

- Understand that transformation is a process, not an instant outcome. Celebrate every small victory and learn from setbacks. Progress is a testament to your dedication.

3. Prioritize Self-Care:

- Self-care is not selfish; it's a fundamental aspect of maintaining balance and well-being. Prioritize self-care as a daily practice, and watch how it transforms your life.

4. Build Resilience:

- Challenges are part of life's journey. Embrace them as opportunities to grow and become more resilient. Your ability to bounce back from adversity is a testament to your inner strength.

5. Share Your Journey:

- As you make progress, consider sharing your experiences and wisdom with others. Your story has the power to inspire and support those who may be seeking similar transformations.

6. Embrace Change:

- Change is inevitable, but it can be a source of growth and renewal. Embrace it with an open heart and a willingness to adapt.

7. Your Well-Being Matters:

- Always remember that your well-being is a priority. You deserve a life filled with peace, happiness, and fulfillment. Never settle for less.

8. Seek Support When Needed:

- Don't hesitate to seek support, whether from loved ones or professionals, when you encounter challenges or need guidance. Asking for help is a sign of strength.

9. Your Journey Continues:

- Your journey towards a stress-free life is an ongoing one. It's marked by continual growth, learning, and self-discovery. Embrace the adventure that lies ahead.

10. The Best is Yet to Come:

As you continue on your path, know that you are not alone. Your determination, courage, and commitment to your well-being are commendable. The transformation you seek is within your reach, and with persistence, you will achieve it.

May your days be filled with peace, joy, and the fulfillment that comes from living a stress-free life. Keep moving forward, for the journey is a beautiful one, and the destination is worth every step.

 Here are some resources that can provide further support and learning on your journey towards a stress-free life:

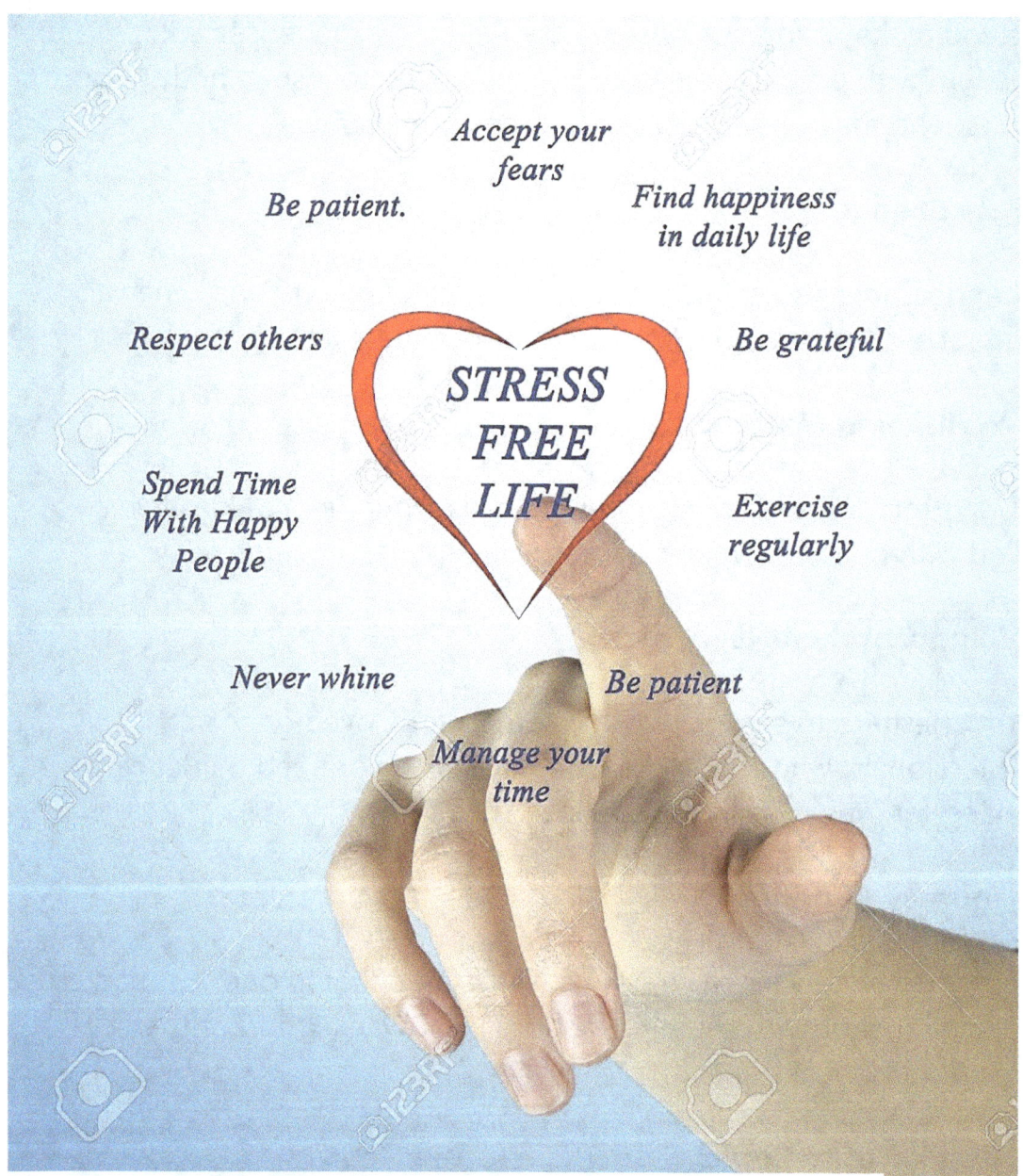

Fig. 12: How stress free life looks like

Books:

1. "The Relaxation and Stress Reduction Workbook" by Martha Davis, Elizabeth Robbins Eshelman, and Matthew McKay.
2. "The Power of Now: A Guide to Spiritual Enlightenment" by Eckhart Tolle - A transformative book on mindfulness and living in the present moment.
3. "Daring Greatly: How the Courage to Be Vulnerable Transforms the Way We Live, Love, Parent, and Lead" by Brené Brown - A guide to embracing vulnerability and building resilience.
4. "Atomic Habits: An Easy & Proven Way to Build Good Habits & Break Bad Ones" by James Clear - Learn how to create positive habits and reduce stress through effective behavior change.

Websites and Apps:

1. **Headspace:** A meditation and mindfulness app with guided sessions for stress reduction.
2. **Calm:** Another popular meditation and relaxation app that offers guided sessions and sleep stories.
3. **Mindful.org:** An online resource for mindfulness practices, articles, and courses.
4. **Psychology Today:** An online platform with articles, expert blogs, and a therapist directory for mental health support.

Online Courses and Workshops:

1. **Coursera:** Offers courses on mindfulness, stress management, and well-being from universities and institutions worldwide.
2. **edX:** Provides courses on psychology, resilience, and related topics from top universities.

Therapy and Counselling:

1. **BetterHelp:** An online platform connecting individuals with licensed therapists for counselling and support.

2. **Talkspace:** Offers online therapy and counselling services for a wide range of mental health concerns.

Support Groups:

1. **Meetup.com:** Search for local or online support groups related to stress management, mindfulness, or personal growth.
2. **SupportGroups.com:** An online community where you can find and join support groups on various topics, including stress and anxiety.

Professional Help:

If you find that stress is significantly impacting your life and well-being, consider seeking support from a mental health professional such as a therapist, counsellor, or psychiatrist. They can provide personalized guidance and treatment options tailored to your needs.

Remember that everyone's journey is unique, and it's important to explore resources and support systems that resonate with you personally. Whether through books, apps, therapy, or community groups, these resources can complement your efforts and provide valuable insights as you continue your pursuit of a stress-free and fulfilling life.

In the appendix of your book on "How to Live a Stress-Free Life," you can include supplementary materials, references, and resources to enhance the reader's experience and understanding. Here are some ideas for what you can include in the appendix:

1. Worksheets and Exercises:

- Provide printable worksheets and exercises related to stress management, self-assessment, and goal setting. These practical tools can help readers apply the concepts discussed in the book to their own lives.

2. Additional Reading Recommendations:

- Create a list of recommended books, articles, and research papers related to stress management, mindfulness, resilience, and other relevant topics. This can serve as a reading list for readers who want to delve deeper into the subject.

3. Mindfulness and Relaxation Resources:

- Offer links to websites, apps, and guided audio resources for mindfulness meditation, deep breathing exercises, and relaxation techniques. Readers can use these resources to practice and reinforce what they've learned.

4. Journaling Prompts:

- Provide journaling prompts to encourage self-reflection and self-awareness. These prompts can help readers explore their thoughts, emotions, and stress triggers.

5. Glossary of Terms:

- Include a glossary that defines key terms and concepts introduced in the book. This can be especially helpful for readers who are new to the subject.

6. Additional Case Studies and Success Stories:

- Share more real-life success stories and case studies of individuals who have overcome stress and found a path to a stress-free life. These stories can serve as inspiration and practical examples.

7. Resources for Seeking Professional Help:

- Offer contact information and guidance on how to find and connect with mental health professionals, therapists, counsellors, or support groups for those who may require professional assistance.

8. Online Communities and Forums:

- Mention online communities and forums where readers can engage with others who are on similar journeys towards stress reduction and well-being. These platforms can provide a sense of belonging and peer support.

9. Acknowledgments:

- Acknowledge and thank individuals, organizations, or experts who contributed to the development of the book or provided valuable insights during the writing process.

Here are some examples of worksheets, templates, and additional resources that you can include in the appendix of your book on "How to Live a Stress-Free Life" to aid and support readers:

1. Stress Assessment Worksheet:

- A self-assessment tool that helps readers identify their stressors, rate their stress levels, and prioritize areas for stress reduction.

2. Weekly Planner Template:

- A blank weekly planner template for readers to use in organizing their schedules, setting priorities, and allocating time for self-care and stress reduction activities.

3. Daily Mindfulness Journal:

- A journal template with prompts for recording daily mindfulness exercises, reflections on stress triggers, and gratitude moments.

4. Goal Setting Worksheet:

- A worksheet to guide readers in setting SMART (Specific, Measurable, Achievable, Relevant, Time-bound) goals related to stress reduction and personal well-being.

5. Breathing Exercises Guide:

- An illustrated guide that explains various deep breathing techniques for stress relief, complete with step-by-step instructions.

6. Sleep Diary Template:

- A sleep diary for tracking sleep patterns and identifying factors that may affect sleep quality. This can help readers improve their sleep hygiene.

7. Positive Affirmations Cards:

- Printable cards with positive affirmations for readers to use as daily reminders to maintain a positive mindset.

8. Self-Care Checklist:

- A checklist of self-care activities and ideas that readers can use to ensure they are regularly engaging in self-nurturing practices.

9. Additional Reading List:

- Check online And Departmental Store.

10. Resource Directory:

- A directory of online and offline resources, including support groups, therapy options, and local community resources that readers can turn to for additional help and guidance.

11. Sample Stress-Reduction Plan:

- A template that guides readers in creating their personalized stress-reduction plan, including goals, strategies, and a timeline for implementation.

12. Gratitude Journal Template:

- A journal template that encourages readers to cultivate gratitude by recording daily moments of thankfulness.

-

Provided Here below is a list of recommended books, websites, and apps for stress management here is a list of recommended books, websites, and apps for stress management.

Books:

1. "The Relaxation and Stress Reduction Workbook" by Martha Davis, Elizabeth Robbins Eshelman, and Matthew McKay.
2. "The Power of Now: A Guide to Spiritual Enlightenment" by Eckhart Tolle - A transformative book on mindfulness and living in the present moment.
3. "Daring Greatly: How the Courage to Be Vulnerable Transforms the Way We Live, Love, Parent, and Lead" by Brené Brown - A guide to embracing vulnerability and building resilience.
4. "Atomic Habits: An Easy & Proven Way to Build Good Habits & Break Bad Ones" by James Clear - Learn how to create positive habits and reduce stress through effective behavior change.
5. "Full Catastrophe Living: Using the Wisdom of Your Body and Mind to Face Stress, Pain, and Illness" by Jon Kabat-Zinn - A comprehensive guide to mindfulness-based stress reduction.

Websites:

1. **Headspace:** A meditation and mindfulness app with guided sessions for stress reduction. (Website: www.headspace.com)
2. **Calm:** Another popular meditation and relaxation app that offers guided sessions and sleep stories. (Website: www.calm.com)

3. **Mindful.org:** An online resource for mindfulness practices, articles, and courses. (Website: www.mindful.org)
4. **Psychology Today:** An online platform with articles, expert blogs, and a therapist directory for mental health support. (Website: www.psychologytoday.com)

Apps:

1. **Headspace:** This app provides guided meditation sessions, mindfulness exercises, and sleep stories to reduce stress and promote well-being.
2. **Calm:** Offers guided meditation, relaxation techniques, and sleep stories to help users manage stress and improve sleep quality.
3. **Insight Timer:** A meditation app with a vast library of free guided meditations, mindfulness courses, and a supportive community.
4. **Breathe2Relax:** An app that teaches deep breathing techniques for stress management and relaxation.
5. **Happify:** Uses science-based activities and games to boost happiness, reduce stress, and build resilience.
6. **Stress and Anxiety Companion:** Offers a variety of tools and resources for managing stress and anxiety, including relaxation exercises and mood tracking.
7. **MyFitnessPal:** Helps users track nutrition, exercise, and sleep patterns, promoting a healthier lifestyle and reducing stress.

These resources can serve as valuable tools for readers looking to further explore stress management techniques, practice mindfulness, and find support in their journey toward a stress-free life.

Acknowledgments

Before we conclude this journey together, I want to take a moment to express my heartfelt gratitude to you, the reader.

Thank you for choosing to embark on the path toward a stress-free life by picking up this book. Your decision to invest time and effort in your well-being is commendable, and it's my sincere hope that the knowledge and insights shared within these pages have proven valuable to you.

I also want to extend my appreciation to the countless individuals, authors, researchers, and experts whose wisdom and contributions have shaped the content of this book.

Your work in the fields of stress management, mindfulness, resilience, and well-being has been instrumental in creating a comprehensive guide for readers seeking a more balanced and fulfilling life.

To my family and friends who have provided unwavering support, encouragement, and patience throughout the writing process, I am deeply grateful.

Your belief in the importance of this work and your understanding of the time and dedication it required have been invaluable.

Lastly, I want to thank the countless readers who have shared their own stories of transformation, resilience, and success. Your experiences have illuminated the path and have been a constant source of inspiration.

As you continue your journey toward a stress-free life,

I wish you an abundance of peace, joy, and contentment.

May your days be filled with self-discovery, growth, and the serenity that comes from embracing a life free from the burdens of chronic stress.

Thank you for allowing me to be a part of your journey, and may you find the happiness and fulfillment you deserve.

With heartfelt gratitude,

Josiah Githinji